JOINT REPLACEMENT
IN THE
UPPER LIMB

JOINT REPLACEMENT
IN THE
UPPER LIMB

I Mech E CONFERENCE PUBLICATIONS 1977-5

Conference sponsored by the
Medical Engineering Section of
The Institution of Mechanical Engineers
and the
British Orthopaedic Association

London, 18-20 April 1977

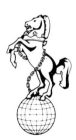

Published by
Mechanical Engineering Publications Limited for
The Institution of Mechanical Engineers
LONDON AND NEW YORK

First published 1977

This volume is complete in itself.

There is no supplementary discussion volume.

ISBN 0 85298 358 1

Made and printed in Great Britain at
The Burlington Press, Foxton, Royston, Hertfordshire.

CONTENTS

SOME SIGNIFICANT ASPECTS OF NORMAL UPPER LIMB FUNCTIONS

PROF. P.R. DAVIS, MB, BS, PhD, FRCS, LRCP, FI Biol
Dept. Human Biology and Health, University of Surry, Guildford

SYNOPSIS The paper starts by comparing the functional adaptations of the upper limb during human evolution with its functional requirements in modern urbanised society. Evolution has resulted in an upper limb well adapted to long distance locomotion and infrequent lifting and handling. Modern society requires frequent manipulation, much enhanced precision activity, and a reduced locomotor need.

A classification of functions relevant to joint replacement is then offered, including:-

> Balance and locomotion
>
> Feeding
>
> Manipulation
>
> Sensory activity
>
> Defence - aggression
>
> Communication
>
> Hygiene

Consideration is then given to the pendular activity and the timing of energy inputs into the free swinging limb during locomotion, and the importance at operation of retaining the normal mass distribution within the limb is emphasised.

Modern use of the upper limb places many demands on its precision activities. A simple test of sensori-motor precision is described, and it is suggested that sensori motor testing should play a more important part in post operative assessment than is sometimes the case. The increasing need for static joint activity is emphasised.

Finally, some observations concerning the ranges and frequencies of joint movements in the upper limb are put forward, dividing these into those deriving from basic living, those from work, and those from leisure activities.

Observations on joint movements frequencies in a number of occupations are presented and their significances are discussed.

INTRODUCTION

May I start by thanking the organisers for extending their invitation to me to give the opening paper at this conference. I am deeply conscious of the honour involved and of the responsibility that derives from it.

I must admit that a review of the programme and of the paper preprints was somewhat daunting, as many of the matters I had though I might consider are already included in better form as contributions from others later in the programme: these include detailed considerations of individual joint mechanisms, so important in designing joint replacements, questions of materials, lubrication and anchorage, and the magnitudes of transarticular forces and their resistances.

However, there are three areas of less immediate import in which I, with some pretensions to biology, can offer some observations which may be of value. These are, firstly, a suggestion that the evolutionary process is worth considering in relation to joint disease; secondly, a classification of normal upper limb functions which may be helpful when considering individual patients requiring surgical implantation procedures; and finally an appraisal of the frequencies and ranges of upper limb movements in a number of different occupations which may affect consideration of the type of joint replacement to be used in an individual case.

Evolutionary aspects

Human history is short lived when compared with the time span required for the evolution of human locomotion. Recent discoveries in Africa and elsewhere show conclusively that Man has been a biped for well over 3.5 million years, a period covered by about 900,000 generations at present reproduction rates. For virtually all of this time Man operated as a nomadic hunter gatherer, having no fixed abode, eating where the food grew or camping by any large kill until it was consumed or became uneatable. Calculations based on the summarisations of Bowles (1974) suggest that throughout this time Man walked for 10 - 70 miles per day, carried virtually nothing except for his (or, perhaps, her) youngest progeny, wore next to no clothing, built minimum shelters on infrequent occasions, made modest stone tools on the spot for hunting and skinning, but discarding them as soon as their immediate purpose had been fulfilled. Thus one can speculate that upper limb usage was mainly locomotor, with short periods of power use for defence, aggression and crude flaying butchery, and more precise use for berry picking, extracting insects from wood and so on. Almost all activities would have been dynamic in nature, static activity being virtually absent. Late in this period the use of projectiles seems to have developed, either as bolas type weapons or for spearing or hamstringing game.

With the number of generations as large as this, quite mild selective forces can be shown to have strong adaptive effects, and the only possible conclusion is that human skeletal mechanisms evolved very well to become nearly perfectly adapted to that mode of life.

As adaptation proceeded, Man became more successful in biological terms, and his population density began to increase significantly. This led to two important consequences, centrifugal migration and selective food shortages.

Migration away from the normal subtropical inhabitation areas has led in turn to a variety of secondary adaptations, such as loss of skin pigmentation, changes in body form, and probably to an as yet unexplored number of minor skeletal variations, which in sum make up the various racial characteristics one sees in different human populations.

The greatest relevant change has been the question of food. The human response to food shortage has been the change from mobility to settlement. Settlement in its turn required the construction of permanent shelters, the storage of food and the disposal of waste, the domestication of animals, the tilling of land and the sowing of seed, the creation and storing of knowledge, and the design of leisure activity.

The timing of this change has varied in different areas, but can perhaps be first seen in embryonic form in Neanderthal Man some 50,000 years ago. The most significant changes towards fully settled life appear but 10,000 years ago at first in the Middle East, where, in the so called fertile crescent from the east Mediterranean litoral across the north of Arabia and into the Tigris valley, primitive agriculture commenced, and has now spread to nearly every part of the inhabited world.

Thus the new environment was only significantly created by Man some 10,000 years ago or less, a period covered by but 400 generations, a number quite insufficient for all but the smallest skeletal adaptations.

Modern Man's skeleton must be regarded as a structure designed for long distance walking, frequent feeding, and infrequent and light load carrying. In contrast, modern western civilis-

ation requires it to be used but little for locomotion, largely for moderate or heavy load carrying and manipulative activities and other needs requiring much static activity, and infrequently (but intensively for short intervals) for feeding. Thus, in determining the design of a replacement joint it may be possible to provide greater adaptation to heavy static loads than exists in the natural state.

Classification of upper limb functions.

I would now like to offer a classification of upper limb functions in the context of joint replacement. The human upper limb can be thought of as having the following main functions, these being those most likely to be affected by joint disorders:

1. Balance and locomotion

2. Feeding

3. Manipulation

4. Sensory activity

5. Defence - aggression

6. Communication

7. Personal hygiene

Feeding, defence, communication and personal hygiene are all important functions in the context of this paper, but their significances seem obvious, and they can perhaps be mentioned as an aide-memoire without further consideration.

Less relevant to todays purposes are the parts the limb plays in contributing to thermo-regulation, fat storage, fluid balance and similar physiological phenomena, and I have excluded these entirely from my present thesis.
LOCOMOTION
With regard to locomotion, when walking the upper limb appears to act in many ways as a pendulum, (Elftman, 1939) and is necessarily affected by physical laws. However, in all but slow walking it departs from pure pendular movement, being actively accelerated from the extended position and actively decelerated as it approaches its limit of flexion. Equally, from flexion it is initially actively accelerated, and again actively decelerated towards its limit of extension. (Dyson, 1967, Ballasteros et al, 1965). The result of this muscular activity is to apply forces at the shoulder which may be resolved into smaller vertical and larger horizontal components.

With the elbow straight, the centre of gravity of the limb as a whole lies in close relationship to the elbow joint, and if one applies the results of anthropometry as applied to walking cyclographs one can use the standard pendulum equations to determine the free swing frequency of the limb, which at slow rates swings from a notional fulcrum in the neck. As stepping rate increases the scapula becomes more fixed, lowering the position of the notional fulcrum and shortening the pendulum. With further increase in step rate the elbow is flexed, thus raising the centre of gravity towards the fulcrum. Thus, progressively, the distance between the notional fulcrum and the centre of gravity of the pendular mass is

2

decreased with increasing stepping rate. Thus preservation of mass distribution is important when replacing substantial portions of the skeleton.

Using this pendular approach, one can determine the theoretical free swinging frequencies of the limb, and compare them with observed behaviour. In observations on six subjects we have obtained consistent figures, and Table I gives a representative result.

Table I Relationship between effective upper limb length and pace rates at different locomotor speeds for 1 subject.

	Fulcrum -CG (cm)	Swing time (sec) $(2\pi\sqrt{l/g})$	Swings per min.	Pace rate Theory	Pace rate Observed
Stroll	30	1.099	54.57	109	98
Walk	24	0.983	61.04	122	120
Trot	21	0.920	65.22	130	128
Run	15	0.777	77.22	154	150+

Thus the mean swing time for locomotion at speeds up to slow running accords well with the free pendulum time, and it seems to be the energy needed to perturb the acceleration due to gravity that is used for locomotor assistance.

Part of this assistance derives largely from the horizontal components of force. As the limb is actively moved from the extended position, an equal and opposite horizontal force pushes that side of the thorax backwards, and as the limb is actively moved backwards from the flexed position, that side of the thorax is moved forwards. With two limbs in reciprocal action, rotatory forces are thus exerted on the upper thorax to oppose the thoracic rotation which would otherwise be caused by lower limb activity. Above slow running speeds, arm swing rates have to be increased markedly above natural pendulum frequencies, and presumably the energy inputs and consequent rotational forces rise markedly with further increases in speed above this level. Since the rotatory damping effect on the thorax is bilaterally symmetrical it would seem important that any replacement should reflect the mass of the removed part as closely as possible.

Sensation and manipulation.

Manipulation is perhaps worthy of greater note, as it is conditioned more largely by minor skeletal changes than some of the other functions. The now classical division of grips by Napier (1956) into power and precision will be familiar, as will the division of the hand in to the three radial digits as being more manipulative and the two ulnar ones as being more gripping (Yamashita and Mori, 1963). Projectile activity is a type of manipulation which is important in many occupations and superficially may be thought of as a separate manual activity, but in fact it falls within these other classifications. In most manipulations, particularly in precision activities, the degree of accuracy is conditioned as much by the proprioceptive and central control of limb movements as by the mechanical integrity of the joints and bones, and it is particularly

on this sensory activity that I would like to comment today.

We have recently carried out some experiments concerned with the accuracy of control of arm positions, by asking subjects to hold a stylus against a target point firstly at full arms reach with the trunk supported, and again with the elbow supported. At full arms stretch in young subjects the stylus remains within about 2mm of the target, angular control at the shoulder being within 0.4°. With the elbow and trunk supported, the mean target error was within 1.2mm of the target, and again the control was of the order of 0.4°. For activity requiring greater precision than this, the hand must be supported close to the target.

Table II Deviations (mm) from point target. (n=16, 30 sec.)

A. At arms length

Horizontal	$\bar{x}$	3.4	σ	0.78
Vertical	$\bar{x}$	4.0	σ	0.75

B. Elbow supported

Horizontal	$\bar{x}$	2.4	σ	0.68
Vertical	$\bar{x}$	2.6	σ	0.85

Thus, when assessing the success of joint replacement, I would like to suggest that a simple target test of this nature is introduced to help assess the functional potential of the treated limb for those persistently engaged in precision activities.

Frequencies of upper limb movements.

Finally, a few observations on frequencies of joint movements may be helpful to those at this conference who have to consider fatigue effects on implanted materials.

One can divide the use of the upper limb in to three groups of activities, namely, those for basic living, those for work, and those for leisure activities. Basic living includes getting up and dressing, personal hygiene, feeding, undressing at night and so on, and in Western civilisation follows a pattern which is generally applicable to the great majority of subjects. Work movements, of course, depend upon individual occupations, as do those deriving from leisure activities.

For basic living I have carried out observations on my own family, in the University refectory and in similar establishments. Thus my sample is a specialised one, but I do not think it would differ greatly in other households. To carry out such observations properly one would need to conduct either extensive goniometry, or a most carefully analysed 3D film. The figures I have obtained come from careful observation of the unwitting, so the angles of movement are as observed, not measured. The frequencies were obtained either by tally counting directly, or by counts off cine films. They do not include purely locomotor activity associated with basic living.

TABLE III. *Estimated number (and ranges in degrees) of joint movements in basic living activities.*

Right arm, Summer (8 males, 1 female)

	Shoulder (Fl. - ext)	Elbow (Fl. - ext)	Pron - Sup.	Wrist (Fl. - ext)	Grips Prec.	Power
Getting up	210 (+40, -30)	330 (130 -0)	400 (+90, -20)	425 (0, -40)	30	28
Breakfast	60 (+30, -0)	75 (130 -80)	55 (+90, -10)	65 (+80,-40)	35	6
Lunch	90 (+30, -0)	140 (130 -40)	100 (+90, -15)	110 (+15,-45)	60	9
Dinner	120 (+30, -0)	180 (130 -0)	130 (+90, -20)	150 (+15,-45)	70	12
To bed	140 (+50, -35)	170 (130 -0)	210 (+90, -20)	310 (0,-40)	16	34
TOTAL	620	895	895	1,100	211	89

Such activities as television watching, crossword solving and the like, together with bathing and going to the lavatory have not been included, so that this total is a considerable underestimate, and one could guess that the basic movement frequency is of the following order:-

TABLE IV *Personal daily basic movement frequency (estimated).*

Shoulder	Elbow	Pron-Sup.	Wrist	Grip Prec.	Power
1000	1400	1400	1800	300	150

The relatively large numbers of precision grips can be taken as giving the relative importance of precision in present day life.

As we saw earlier, in general basic locomotor activity has declined from a daily average of between 10 and 70 miles in pre-Neolithic times, and it now seems to be of the order of 2 - 4 miles a day with very little running. So one can add an estimate of some 2,500+ shoulder swings (20-10°) with slight movements of the elbow (15-0°) of the same order of frequency, giving a total base frequency of 3,500 for the shoulder and 4,000+ for the elbow.

When it comes to occupation, then things become difficult. However, my team have kindly looked at our records for certain occupations which lend themselves to this approach. Where a job is regularly repetitive one can determine the mean number of movements per cycle and multiply this by the number of cycles per day to give an approximation of the total number of movements. Using this approach they have obtained the data shown in Table V.

One of the most extensive examples of repetitive movement is that of the copy typist (Table V1), whose movements when typing consist of slight finger and wrist flexion for each symbol typed, with larger less frequent movements when changing the paper and similar needs.

TABLE VI *Frequency of movements in a working day, copy typing.*

Symbols typed	100,000 - 190,000
Key pressure	65 - 110 gm.
Key movement	5 - 11 mm.

Thus we can get some sort of estimate for a working individual. For many, movements run in the tens of thousands per day, and for some this may be in the hundred thousands. Loads per movement differ widely, from the few grammes of the typist to the many kilogrammes of the builders labourer.

Finally, returning to my opening remarks, it is interesting to consider the pre-Neolithic rates in comparison. Blurton-Jones (1976) has recently studied nomadic Bushwoman in the field, it being the female who does most of the manual work in the Kalahari desert. At the end of the dry season the average Bushwoman walks 12-18 miles per day, gathers and processes about 400 nuts, and may lift and lower her child some 20 times. Thus her manual activity, with concomitant arm movements, is less than 1,000 per day, but her locomotor movements of the order of 12,000 arm swings are much increased compared with modern society.

TABLE V. *Frequency of movements during the working day.*

	Shoulder (Fl. ext)	Elbow (Fl. ext.)	Pron/Sup.	Wrist (Fl. ext.)	Grip Prec.	Power
Bricklayer (Laying hand)	5,700 +55 -45	3,800 90 0	3,800 +45 -45	3,800 -5 +15		1,900
Wallplasterer (float hand)	7,800 +80 -50	5,200 150 -0	3,900 +70 +30	5,800 -		600
Scaffolder (preferred hand)	1,100 +80 -20	1,100 100 -0	-	-	120	400
Labourer (site stacking)	6,200 +45 -0	8,800 90 -0	4,400 +40 -0	4,400 0 -30		4,400

4

CONCLUSIONS

Thus I would like to suggest firstly that, when considering upper limb joint replacement in the Western world one should remember that one is concerned with a joint designed in Nature for one or a few thousand dynamic movements per day which may be _performing_ movement frequencies of at least one and perhaps even two orders higher, and that many of these movements may have a large static component. It may thus be possible to better Nature as far as joint surface performance is concerned.

Secondly, while motor performance is commonly used as a measure of post operative success, may I suggest that sensori-motor activity is perhaps more relevant when considering upper limb activity, and a simple battery of sensori-motor tests might usefully be applied to all post operative patients.

As a consequence of this I would like to enter a plea to suggest that preservation of neural feed back mechanisms is so important for the upper limb that it must be made a major consideration for anyone designing or inserting joint replacements.

REFERENCES

Ballasteros,M.L.F., Buchthal, F and Rosenfalck,P. The pattern of muscular activity during the arm swing of natural walking.
     Acta Physiol.Scand., _63_, 296-310, 1965

Blurton Jones, A. Personal communication.

Bowles, S. Dissertation, University of Surrey, 1970.

Dyson, G. The mechanics of athletics. University of London Press, 1967.

Elftman, H. The functions of the arm in walking.
     Hum. Biol, _11_, 529-535, 1939.

Napier, J.R. The prehensile movements of the human hand.
     J.Bone Jt. Surg., _38-B_, 902-913,1956.

Yamashita, T. and Mori, M. Engineering approaches to function of fingers. Report Inst.
     Indust.Sci., U.Tokyo. _13_, 60-110, 1963.

C150/77

THE DESIGN OF A METAL-TO-METAL TOTAL SHOULDER JOINT PROSTHESIS

V.H. WHEBLE, MA,BM,BCh,FRCS,DTM
Tameside General Hospital, Ashton under Lyne

J.SKORECKI, BSc, MSc, PhD, DSc, C.Eng, FIMechE and
G. THOMPSON, MSc
Department of Mechanical Engineering, University of Manchester
Institute of Science and Technology

SYNOPSIS Experience gained from titanium humerus head replacement has led to an all-metal total shoulder ball-and-socket design permitting full articulation and resistance to pull. Consideration of wear on the articulating surfaces and compatibility with bone resulted in combining cobalt-chromium with titanium.

INTRODUCTION

1.   In 1963 one of the authors was faced with the problem of treating a severe shatter fracture of the upper end of the humerus, with considerable displacement of the head fragments. Neer's (ref. 1) prosthesis was not available and the only other acceptable design of humeral head prosthesis was of Jackson Burrows (ref. 2), also not obtainable. A new prosthesis was designed based on the Jackson Burrows prosthesis and subsequently modified to make production by a manufacturer feasible. This prosthesis was made of titanium and has been used for the treatment of shatter fractures of the humeral head, and other conditions, up to the present time.

The main differences between the Wheble and the Jackson Burrows prostheses were the shaping of the neck portion of the stem, as well as the taper and section of the stem itself. The shaping of the entrance and exit of the holes in the head was modified to make the passage of a needle easier (see Fig. 1). It was also necessary to design right and left-handed versions. The manufacturers found it easier to produce this prosthesis from a casting by finishing techniques rather than by milling from bar stock. The stem was treated by etching, using the 250 grain-size glass-bead technique, while the head was polished to a mirror finish. When satisfactorily fixed in place there has been very little evidence of any reaction between the prosthesis and the bone and the bond became sound within a matter of weeks; no evidence of loosening has been found with the passage of time.

The information gained by the use of this humeral head prosthesis has been incorporated in the development of the Wheble-Skorecki total shoulder prosthesis.

2.   THE INDICATION FOR SHOULDER ARTHROPLASTY

Experience with the humeral head prosthesis has resulted from its use in five groups of conditions.

(1)   Shatter fractures of the head of the humerus

This type of fracture was first described by Codman in 1934 (ref. 3); it is characterised by separation of the humeral head from the shaft and tuberosities and shattering of the head itself. Parts of the head may be displaced through tears in the shoulder capsule. Some fragments may escape through gaps between the muscles of the rotator cuff, which have retracted with small fragments of the humerus attached. The greater tuberosity tends to retract upwards under the acromial arch, while the lesser tuberosity is pulled forwards and upwards under the coracoid process. The lesser tuberosity fragment is frequently 'V' shaped and includes part of the bicipital groove, so that the biceps tendon lies in the gap between the shattered fragments. In all, there may be as many as eight fragments and reconstruction is impossible, as the head fragments have lost their blood supply.

(2)   Failed reconstruction operations of the
       McLaughlin or Codman type

Suturing of the tuberosities to the head and shaft of the humerus, repair of the biceps tendon and the deltoid without repair of the shoulder capsule has been a standard procedure for such fractures since it was recommended by Codman (ref. 3). The modified procedure of McLaughlin (ref. 4) in which the subscapularis is interposed between the damaged head and the glenoid has also been recommended. Experience has shown that these procedures have not proved uniformly successful and in particular, where the blood supply of the head has been affected, a painful stiff shoulder results.

(3)   Rheumatoid arthritis of the shoulder

Rheumatoid arthritis of the shoulder is a destructive disease in which the synovial lining and capsule become damaged, as well as the head itself. As the rotator cuff muscles are intimately bound down to the capsule, they also become involved at their insertions and holes appear through which the head may displace. Displacement upwards, if the supraspinatus is involved, produces the condition described by Lettin (ref. 5) as superior migration of the humerus. Displacement may also take place forwards or backwards, and the surface of the humerus and glenoid may be eroded. Humeral head arthroplasty may not be successful in such cases and, indeed, may prove to be impossible.

(4)   Benign and malignant tumours of the humerus
       at the upper end

Benign and malignant tumours, such as chondroma or slow growing chondro-sarcomata, can be subjected to this operation if they have not invaded the cuff muscles.

(5) Osteoarthritis of the shoulder

Though this is relatively unusual at the shoulder joint, it can occur as a result of the malunion of severe fractures of the humeral head; the loss of joint space and the formation of osteophytes produce severe restriction of gleno-humeral movement, so that only excision of the head and the insertion of a prosthesis is likely to restore movement.

In all these five conditions there are cases where it seems that a more satisfactory solution would require replacement of both the humeral and the glenoid articular surfaces, but humeral head replacement has been the first essential step in developing a total shoulder replacement and has given reasonably satisfactory results.

3. THE OPERATION OF HUMERAL-HEAD REPLACEMENT USING THE WHEBLE PROSTHESIS

The approach follows the standard pattern, a sabre cut incision on the front of the shoulder. In the case of a severe multi-fragment fracture dislocation of the humeral head, the exposure reveals the extent of the problem. When dead portions of the head have been removed, the Wheble humeral-head prosthesis can be fitted into the shaft after reaming the medullary cavity, and the small bone fragments can be sutured round the prosthetic head. This reconstruction of the humerus produces a satisfactory functional humerus, the dislocation can be reduced, the rotator cuff muscles repaired and the deltoid restored to its normal place. The Rowley Bristow procedure (refs. 6,7) using the coracoid process, can be carried out if there is evidence of an anterior capsular tear which could lead to recurrent dislocation. After-care consists of a period of immobilisation, varying from case to case, followed by physiotherapy and occupational therapy.

4. THE RESULTS OF A WHEBLE HUMERAL HEAD REPLACEMENT ARTHROPLASTY

This operation has been performed by various surgeons and the results have been recorded in Tables I and II (see Appendix). As may be seen, there is a general improvement in the degree of pain encountered when the arthroplasty cases are compared with the controls. There is also a general improvement in movements following arthroplasty. These results are comparable with those recorded by Neer (ref. 8) and it seems therefore that the results, though indicating that humeral head replacement is a worthwhile operation, do require an attempt to improve the design.

Comparison of these cases with the controls, including 22 cases of severe fracture of the humeral head and neck, treated in various ways, and one case of rheumatoid arthritis treated by exploration with a view to humeral head replacement without successful completion of the operation, shows that the humeral head replacement was a more satisfactory procedure in every respect. (See Table II).

5. ANALYSIS OF FACTORS INVOLVED IN FAILURE TO REGAIN SHOULDER MOVEMENTS

Unlike the hip joint, the shoulder joint is used for prehension and its chief function is to make possible grasping movements within a wide arc of movement. This is achieved by scapulo-humeral and thoraco-scapular articulations. McConail (ref. 9) has demonstrated that there are also built-in features of movement of the humerus on the scapula whereby rotation also takes place with the simple movements of forward flexion and abduction allowing the humerus to be elevated parallel with the side of the head. The integration of the scapulo-humeral and scapular movements is complex and requires perfect co-ordination of the rotator cuff muscles with those that raise the arm from the side and those that fix and move the scapula. Thus full movement can only be regained after damage and disruption of the bone and musculature if the muscles can be restored perfectly to their normal position and function.

6. DETERMINATION OF THE NORMAL SCAPULO-HUMERAL ARTICULATION

A small sample test has been carried out with a mechanical rig of the range of scapulo-humeral articulation (see Fig. 2). The subjects were all seated on a horizontal hard seat with their spines contacting at two points a vertical bar; the position of the jugular notch of the sternum was monitored with a delicate beam swivelling in a fixed fulcrum while its two ends contacted both the notch and a fixed vertical reference line respectively. Additional checks on the posture of the subject were kept by the experimenter and also by the subject who could see himself in a mirror parallel to his frontal plane. Simultaneous readings were taken of the positions of the two epicondyles of the humerus and of three subcutaneous features on the scapula. The position of the epicondyles was measured by means of a simple pointer giving direct readings in a Cartesian reference frame. The positions of the three points on the scapula were obtained by measuring nine distances (three from each point on the scapula) to nine points in the fixed reference frame.

From these positions the two spherical angles, the longitude and the latitude, of the axis of the humerus were determined for eight evenly spaced peripheral locations of the humerus. These can be visualised as points on a spherical surface forming a continuous 'coastline' enclosing the full range of articulation (see Fig. 3). On reaching each such location the subject was asked to move his arm towards his body as far as he could without discomfort or change of posture. In addition, at each point on the coastline the fullest possible rotation of the arm about the axis of the humerus was measured.

The results of these tests will be used for finding the best possible compromise between the required range of articulation and the wear-strength characteristics of the prosthesis.

The choice of a purely mechanical apparatus was made partly in order to avoid the need of many exposures of the subjects to X-rays as would be required to establish a sufficiently continuous 'coastline' and partly due to the expected difficulty in interpreting the experimental data. The method used lends itself to easy checks and to indefinite 're-sits' of the subjects. The most expensive single item in the apparatus is an average quality photographic camera.

7. THE DESIGN CRITERIA FOR A TOTAL SHOULDER JOINT REPLACEMENT

In certain cases the removal of the capsule of the scapulo-humeral joint and the rotator cuff muscles may be necessary. This can only be done if it were possible to design a total shoulder joint prosthesis to take the place of the rotator cuff and the capsule. It would only be justified initially in those cases where the capsule is already partly destroyed, as in rheumatoid arthritis or by tumours, or has become so fibrotic as to be a barrier to movements of the scapulo-humeral joint such as cases where the Codman and McLaughlin procedures have been attempted and failed. If it was proved to be successful in such cases there would possibly be a case to be made out for total shoulder joint replacement in the treatment of shatter fracture dislocations.

The design criteria needed for a total shoulder joint replacement are thus:-

(i) The joint must be made of materials with especially satisfactory wear characteristics so as to eliminate the need for revision or, if this is not possible, a replaceable bearing should be used so that the scapular and humeral components need not be disturbed once they have been fixed.

(ii) Fixation must be secure and performed with such inert materials that there could be no foreseeable reaction to disturb it.

(iii) The method of fixation must be as simple as possible from the technical point of view.

(iv) Dislocation or fracture of the prosthesis must be resisted or, if it does take place, the bearing of the prosthesis must be replaceable.

(v) If the prosthesis has to be removed, a salvage operation to stabilise the shoulder joint, even at the expense of loss of movement, must be possible.

8. DISCUSSION OF EXISTING TOTAL SHOULDER REPLACEMENT PROSTHESES

Total shoulder joint replacement as a solution to the many problems outlined above has been investigated by a number of workers. Papers on this subject have been published by Lettin and Scales (5), Monteleone (10), Neer (8), Suire (11) and Beddow (12) and all these authors agree that arthroplasty of the shoulder, however it is performed, is pain relieving, but the achievement of satisfactory movement is a hit and miss affair. Lettin has endeavoured, in cases of superior migration, to keep the head of the humerus down far enough to allow abduction of the scapulo-humeral joint to occur. His solution has, however, resulted in restriction of scapulo-humeral abduction and forward flexion. He has also encountered difficulties in achieving satisfactory fixation to the scapula. Reeves has considered a number of different solutions to the problem, involving on the one hand the introduction of a double joint with a ball and socket at each end of a central member and also a ball with a stem fixed

to the scapula articulating with the socket fixed to the humerus. He favours a high density polyethylene liner inside a chromium-cobalt molybdenum alloy retaining socket for the humerus. The scapular component is fixed with pegs and cement as has been done by Lettin at Stanmore.

9. THE MECHANICAL FEATURES OF THE WHEBLE-SKORECKI TOTAL SHOULDER JOINT PROSTHESIS

The design criteria outlined in this paper have been used to develop a metal-to-metal total shoulder joint prosthesis and it will become apparent that the present solution to the problem, based on the previous experience of humeral head replacement, though similar in basic principles to one of the Reeves solutions, has many important new features.

Choice of materials

Because of its known affinity to bone, titanium was again chosen (ref. 13) for the stem of the humeral component, and also for the scapular component and the fixing screws, thus discarding acrylic cement which is known to be somewhat variable in its reactions with bone and particularly when subjected to tensile forces (ref. 14). But, as titanium does not produce a satisfactory articulation with itself and tends to bind, the choice left for the articulating components is between high density polyethylene and chromium-cobalt-molybdenum alloy or an all metal joint between chromium-cobalt molybdenum alloy components. However, high density polyethylene was discarded for the following reason: it has a low tensile strength compared with metals and thus is unable to withstand the tensile forces calculated as acting on the articular component, resulting in hoop and shear stress in the lip of the overlap; this might result in a catastrophic change of the original geometry. It was therefore decided to make the articular components of chromium-cobalt-molybdenum alloy on both sides. It follows from the work of E.G.C. Clarke and J. Hickman (ref.15) that coupling titanium with chromium-cobalt alloys is permissible as regards any possible electro-chemical action in the body.

The problem of carcinogeneic properties of chromium-cobalt alloys when rubbed down to particulate size appears to be exaggerated. The experiments done on laboratory animals (ref. 16) used quantities of this material of proportions unlikely to be reached in a life time of use in the human body.

Fixation

As regards the humeral component, its design features will incorporate applicable, useful features of the Wheble humeral head prosthesis. The design of a scapular component requires new solutions. It is beset by problems. In the authors' prosthesis the scapular component is designed to be fitted with minimal removal of bone. The retaining screws will be inserted into the strong bars of bone that run towards (a) the coracoid process, (b) the scapular spine, and (c) downwards into the strong border of the scapula. In addition, provision is being made for a possible introduction of a screw to run through an anterior lip on the scapular component to fix the small portion of the coracoid with its attached muscles

into the front of the scapula and at the same time
to help stabilise the scapular component. The
fifth point of fixation is a hole of slightly
larger diameter in the glenoid plate which takes
the stem of the scapular articulating component.
The stem is prevented from rotation by the screw
passing from front to back of the glenoid.

The range of movement

The dishlike form of the humeral component
with its small socket makes possible retention of
the ball with the minimum loss of range of movement as it encloses only 18° of arc of the ball
beyond its equator. The boundary of articulation
is reached when contact between the two components
is made outside their spherical surfaces. This
contact is placed as far away as possible from the
centre of the ball and socket so as to reduce the
magnitude of the forces resisting an applied couple.
Thus the rim of the dish rolls on the conical
surface of the stem of the ball rather than making
contact near the neck of the stem at its junction
with the ball.

The solution requires relatively accurately
defined profiles of the two conical surfaces.
Whilst one of the cones, say that of the stem,
will be produced by straight-line generators, the
generator of the dish will be slightly curved so
that under the normal load the contact due to the
Hertzian deflection will take place over a significantly large area but will be separated from the
neck of the stem by a gap increasing gradually
towards the neck. As a consequence, rolling of
the two elements on each other should tend to
promote an inwards flow of lubricant.

Thus, the authors' prosthesis has been
designed to fulfil all the five design criteria
outlined above.

10. IMPLANTATION OF THE BEARING PART OF THE PROSTHESIS

The bearing part of this prosthesis attached
to a special humeral stem and acromial attachment
has already been inserted by A.J. Wilkinson into
a patient with a flail joint after removal of a
tumour. The result is reported to be satisfactory
(see Fig. 5).

ACKNOWLEDGEMENTS

The authors wish to acknowledge the help
which they have received from the late Mr. J.
Flowett, Professors W. Johnson and S.S. Gill,
Mr. Maurice Down, Mr. P. Ferarrio, Mr. A.K.
Akiwumi, Mr. R. Wells, Mr. H. Hamilton, Mr. G.
Sanderson, Mr. G. Biggs, Mrs. Jean Walton, Mrs.
M. Kelsall, Mrs. S. Moss, Mr. J. Howe, the
numerous assistants and the very patient subjects.

For patenting the prosthesis and for the
sustained support, the authors thank the National
Research and Development Corporation and in
particular their Dr. B. C. Patterson for his
unfailing interest and help.

REFERENCES

1. NEER C.S. Articular replacement for humeral
head, J. Bone & Joint Surg., 1955, 37A, 315.

2. BURROWS H.J. Replacement of bone by internal
prostheses, J. Bone & Joint Surg., 1954, 36B, 694.

3. CODMAN E.A. The shoulder. Rupture of the
supraspinatus tendon and other lesions in or about
the subacromial bursa, 1934, (Privately printed).

4. McLAUGHLIN H.L. (Editor), Trauma, 1959,
(W.B. Saunders & Co., Philadelphia).

5. LETTIN A.W.F. and SCALES T.J. Total
replacement of the shoulder joint (two cases),
Proc. Roy. Soc. Med., April 1972, 65, 373-4.

6. HELFET A.S. Coracoid transplantation for
removing dislocation of shoulder, J. Bone & Joint
Surg., 1958, 40B, 198-202.

7. LOMBARDO S.J., KERLAN R.K., JOBE F.W.,
CARTER V.S., BLAZINA M.E. and SHIELDS C.L.
The modified Bristow procedure for recurrent
dislocation of the shoulder, J. Bone & Joint
Surg., March 1976, 58A, 2, 256-261.

8. NEER C.S. Displaced proximal humeral
fractures, Parts I & II, J. Bone & Joint Surg.,
1970, 52A, 1077-1088 and 1089-1103.

9. McCONAILL M.A. Movements of bones and
joints; the significance of shape, J. Bone &
Joint Surg., 1953, 35B, 290-7.

10. MONTELEONE M. L'endoprotesi sostitutiva
nella terapia della fratture-lussazioni dell'
estremita superiore dell'omero', Chir. Organi
Mov., June 1969, 57, 404-11.

11. SUIRE P. Reflexions au sujet de l'anatomie
patholgique et du traitement des fractures
luxations de l'épaule, Chirurgie, Nov. 1970, 96,
918-28.

12. BEDDOW F.H. Shoulder replacement, Proc.
Roy. Soc. Med., March 1970, 69, No. 3.

13. BURROWS H.J., WILSON J.N. and SCALES J.T.
Excision of tumours of humerus and femur with
restoration by internal prostheses, J. Bone &
Joint Surg. (Br), 1975, 57(2), 148-159.

14. CHARNLEY J. Acrylic cement in orthopaedic
surgery, 1970 (E. & S. Livingstone, Edinburgh
and London).

15. CLARKE E.G.C. and HICKMAN J. Investigations
into correlation between electrical potentials of
metals and their behaviour in biological fluids,
J. Bone & Joint Surg., 1953, 35B, 467.

16. HEATH J.C., FREEMAN M.A. and SWANSON S.A.V.
Carcinogenic properties of wear particles from
prostheses made in cobalt-chromium alloy, Lancet,
20 March 1971, 1, 564-6.

APPENDIX

RESULTS OF WHEBLE HUMERAL HEAD REPLACEMENT

TABLE I

Wheble Humeral Head Replacement

Pre-operative diagnosis
4 segment fracture-dislocation	9
Failed Codman reconstruction	3
Chondrosarcoma of humerus	2
Rheumatoid arthritis	1
	15

Control cases

Fractures of humeral head and neck requiring open reduction	5
Fractures of humeral head and neck treated by manipulative reduction	16
Fractures of humeral head and neck requiring arthrodesis	1
Rheumatoid arthritis (failed insertion of prosthesis)	1
	23

TOTAL   38

TABLE II

Results of 15 cases of humeral head replacement
compared with controls, based on gradings for
pain and movement

	Pain Grade I*	II	III	IV	Totals
Grade A**					
H.H.R.	1	0	0	0	1
Control	0	0	0	0	0
Grade B					
H.H.R.	5	1	1	0	7
Control	0	3	0	0	3
Grade C					
H.H.R.	4	1	0	0	5
Control	1	7	4	0	12
Grade D					
H.H.R.	2	0	0	0	2
Control	2	3	2	1	8

*Grade I No pain
Grade II Slight pain only on movements
Grade III Some pain at rest, made worse by
movements
Grade IV Pain constantly present preventing use
of the arm

**Grade A Movement. Full range
Grade B Movement. Loss of less than ½ range
Grade C   Loss of more than ½ range
Grade D Movement. No humero-scapular movement

H.H.R. = Humeral Head Replacement

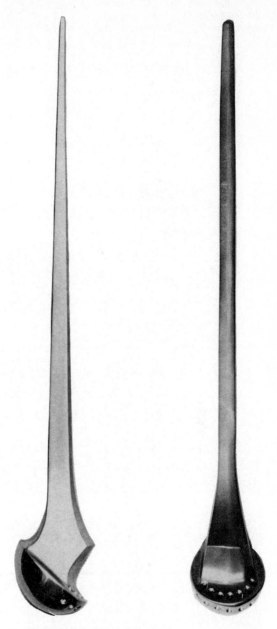

Fig. 1: Wheble humeral head prosthesis

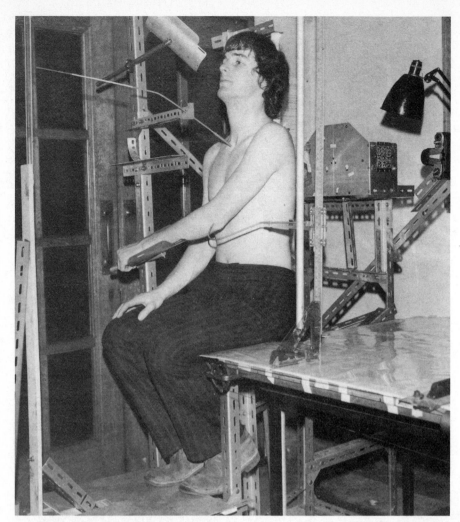

Fig. 2: Scapulo-humeral articulation measuring apparatus

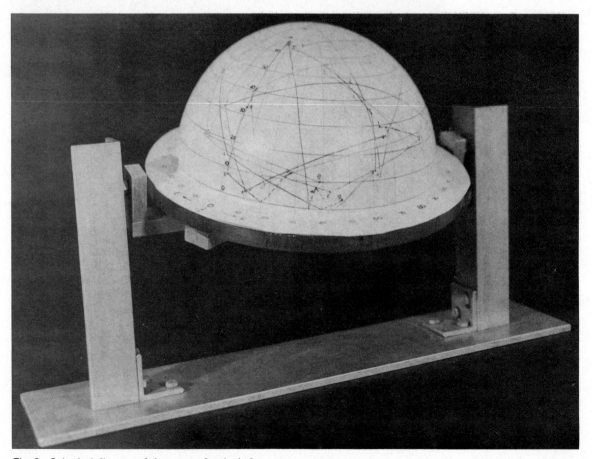

Fig. 3: Spherical diagram of the range of articulation

12

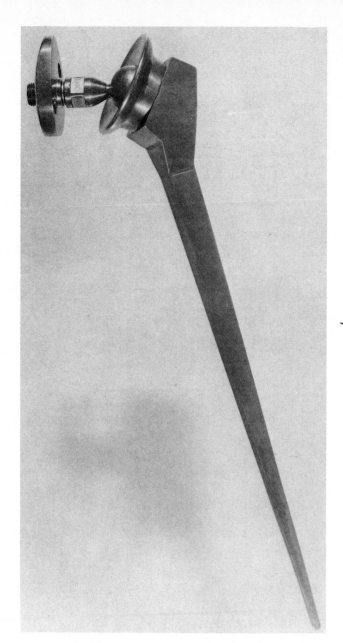

Fig. 4: Wheble-Skorecki prothesis (as inserted in a cadaver)

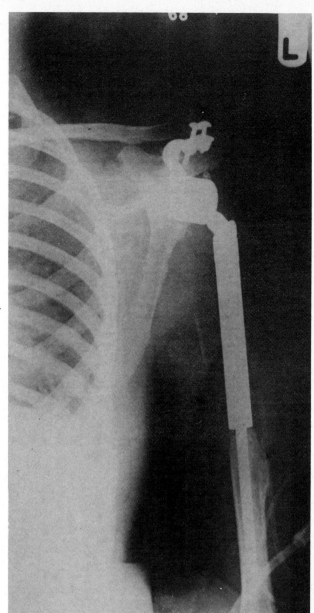

Fig. 5: Prosthesis inserted in a patient in Southampton

14

THE BICKEL GLENOHUMERAL ARTHROPLASTY

R.H. COFIELD, MD, and R.N. STAUFFER, MD
Department of Orthopedics, Mayo Clinic and Mayo Foundation, Rochester, Minnesota, USA

SYNOPSIS   Clinical trials with a fully constrained glenohumeral prosthesis were carried out in 12 patients. The goals established for this type of surgical reconstruction were not achieved with any consistency. Most of the complications were due to mechanical limitations of the design.

INTRODUCTION

1. Some patients with diseases of the glenohumeral joint require a surgical procedure primarily for pain relief and secondarily for better function by increasing their strength, augmenting their motion, or placing their arm in a more useful position. The joint diseases usually result from degenerative or noninfectious inflammatory arthritis or are the residual of old trauma. They most frequently occur in persons of middle age or older.

2. Treatment alternatives previously have been limited to resectional arthroplasty, arthrodesis, or prosthetic humeral head replacement. Resectional procedures, as described by Jones (ref. 1), may relieve pain but such relief has been unpredictable. Strength generally is adequate when the extremity is at the side; however, active motion above the horizontal position is never achieved. Glenohumeral arthrodesis has been successful in paralytic patients (ref. 2). After arthrodesis for arthritic or traumatic conditions, we and others (ref. 3) have been surprised to find that pain relief is often inadequate, restoration of strength is not consistent, and the motion provided by the remaining articulations of the shoulder girdle is often less than required to accomplish easily daily activities. Prolonged postoperative immobilization is necessary, which is particularly undesirable in elderly people. Hemiprosthetic replacement, that is, replacement of the proximal humerus, has been effective in the acute treatment of proximal humeral fractures and osteoarthritis (ref. 4,5). Results are variable in rheumatoid arthritis, being strongly affected by the level of disease activity and the degree of capsular-muscle cuff stability that can be achieved (ref. 6). Rehabilitation is always difficult after proximal humeral prosthetic replacement.

3. Dissatisfaction with these treatment alternatives prompted Dr. William Bickel to develop a glenohumeral prosthesis. The operation was performed to relieve pain and secondarily to provide stability and allow enough motion to accomplish daily activities without the necessity for prolonged immobilization or extensive rehabilitation.

Design parameters

4. The nature of the shoulder joint disease seemed to dictate that both the glenohumeral articular surface and the stabilizing capsular-muscle cuff be replaced by the prosthesis. This would require an articulated joint that was mechanically stable by virtue of its design. In deciding whether to design for mobility or stability, stability was favored. It was decided that 30° or more of glenohumeral prosthetic motion (complemented by motion of the remaining components of the shoulder girdle) would be sufficient to perform comfortably the activities of daily living. Anatomic constraints placed on design are both bony and ligamentous. The small amount of bone available for fixation in the glenoid of the scapula is the most limiting feature. To achieve secure fixation, the glenoid component of the prosthesis needed to be completely contained within the bone of the scapula so that the prosthesis-bone interface area would be maximal and an undesirable moment arm would not be introduced.

5. The selection of prosthetic material was based on previous favorable experience in other areas (for example, total hip and total knee arthroplasties). A metal (stainless steel or chromium-cobalt alloy) with a low friction to polyethylene-bearing surface was selected, and methylmethacrylate was chosen for the prosthesis-bone fixation.

6. Theoretic analysis by Inman et al. indicated that forces in the shoulder reach a maximum at 90° of elevation (ref. 7). At this position, compressive forces against the glenoid are 10.2 times the weight of the extremity or are approximately equal to body weight. Reeves et al. have outlined the biomechanical requirements of a total shoulder prosthesis (ref 8). They concluded that a stable arc of movement of 360° is necessary, that the prime movers should act on the joint in the absence of the stabilizing effect from the rotator cuff musculature, and that the prosthesis should withstand tensile loading of 31.8 to 36.3 kg and a sheer force of 2,073 kg-cm.

7. The prosthesis consisted of a chromium-cobalt humeral component with a spherical head in two sizes, 8 and 10 mm (Fig. 1). The humeral stem was fixed in the medullary canal of the humerus

with methylmethacrylate. The humeral prosthetic head articulated with two high-density polyethylene hemispheres that had a minimal thickness slightly greater than 2 mm. A chromium-cobalt unit encased the head, with its high-density polyethylene socket, and held the components securely together. The outside diameter of the enclosing unit was 18 mm; this was small enough to be contained within the echolocated scapular glenoid. The range of motion was 34° for the 8-mm head and 33° for the 10-mm head.

Mechanical testing

8. Prosthetic resistance to tension and bending load configurations were calculated, using 7.752 x 10^3 kg/cm² as the ultimate tensile strength of cast chromium-cobalt. The head-neck junction of the humeral component was selected as the site for prosthetic failure. In the prosthesis with the 8-mm head, the narrowest portion of the neck was 3 mm. In the 10-mm head prosthesis, the narrowest neck was 4 mm. Calculated tension to failure was 548 kg for the 3-mm neck and 974 kg for the 4-mm neck. Lateral bending to failure occurred at a moment of 20.3 kg-cm for the 3-mm neck and 48.8 kg-cm for the 4-mm neck. With the humeral stem fixed and a force directed against the central portion of the prosthetic head parallel to the axis of the shaft, a force of 67.7 kg was calculated to cause prosthetic neck fracture for the smaller prosthesis, and a force of 122.1 kg was calculated to cause failure of the larger prosthesis. Mechanical bench tests were performed by Dr. Edmund Chao (Orthopedic Biomechanics Laboratory) on six prostheses (Table 1). The load necessary for prosthetic pullout was 62.5 kg on the one 10-mm prosthesis tested. Lateral bending was tested on one 8-mm prosthesis, with moment and load to failure higher than the calculated value. Four tests of bending dislocation were done. Dislocation occurred in only one prosthesis; this occurred at 97.7 kg of load applied. Yielding or fracture of the neck occurred in the other three samples. Testing results varied considerably. Cyclic bending tests were not carried to completion, and no tests were performed to determine the characteristics of the prosthetic-cement or cement-bone junctions.

CLINICAL MATERIAL

9. Twelve patients (six men and six women) underwent the surgical procedure between November 1972 and January 1975. Their ages averaged 60 years and ranged from 44 to 72 years. Four of the patients had the operation on their dominant upper extremity and eight had it on their nondominant upper extremity. Follow-up evaluation averaged 28 months and ranged from 18 to 39 months. The diagnoses were traumatic arthritis (six patients), primary osteoarthritis (five patients), and a painful Neer humeral head prosthesis (one patient). Six patients had undergone previous shoulder surgery (three capsular repairs; one an open reduction with fixation of the fracture; one a cheilotomy; and one a Neer prosthetic replacement with partial acromionectomy).

10. All 12 patients had severe pain preoperatively. The pain characteristically was present at rest, accentuated with use, and bothersome at night. The primary aim of surgery was pain relief

in all 12, with a secondary goal of increasing motion in 5. Five patients had moderate instability at the glenohumeral joint on passive manipulation. Five had mild, five had moderate, and two had severe weakness on muscle testing. Averages of preoperative active shoulder girdle motions are shown in Table 2. Humeral subluxation was noted on preoperative roentgenograms of seven patients (five in an upward direction and two in a downward direction). Glenohumeral joint space narrowing was noted in 10 patients. Seven patients had associated subchondral bone cysts, and eight had marginal osteophytes. Eight patients had significant tuberosity deformities.

11. The surgical technique employed an incision and dissection anteriorly through the deltopectoral interval. The subscapularis tendon was divided and retracted medially. Bone was removed from the medullary canal of the humerus and the glenoid process of the scapula. The humeral prosthesis was cemented in 30° of retroversion. The humeral head was then placed in the high-density polyethylene hemispheres, and the enclosing unit was slipped over the hemispheres. This complex was then cemented into the glenoid cavity. The operation was often extremely difficult, particularly in the post-traumatic patients. Glenoid fractures were produced during prosthetic placement in four patients. Repeat glenoid placements were necessary in four patients (because of poor fixation in three and dislocation at the operation in one). Two patients had the glenoid component fixation supplemented with chromium-cobalt mesh. The condition of the rotator cuff was noted in six patients: it was intact in five and torn in one.

12. Complications occurred during the early part of the series and were often associated with the placement of the 8-mm humeral head (Table 3). This size prosthesis was used in three patients. The first patient had a bony fracture at surgery. Three glenoid placements were necessary, the last being supplemented with mesh. At 6 months, the glenoid component with its cement was dislodged from the scapula. The patient's symptoms began after swinging a golf club. He had a successful arthrodesis using autogenous bone grafts from the ilium on the second attempt. The second patient had no operative complication but at 8 months, while rolling in bed, he fractured the humeral neck of the prosthesis. Replacement without problems was accomplished with the larger prosthesis. The third patient needed two glenoid placements because of dislocation at operation. At 3 weeks, dislocation occurred again. A 10-mm prosthesis was reinserted. The patient did well for 38 months, at which time the prosthetic humeral neck fractured. He has subsequently had a resectional arthroplasty. All of the complications have been or are potentially salvageable. The need for a second operation did not seem to jeopardize the final result. The eighth patient in our series had no operative problems, but at 1 week, the glenoid component dislodged. It was replaced, the fixation being supplemented with mesh. The patient has had no subsequent problems. All of the complications have been, or are potentially, salvageable.

13. Clinical follow-up involved 11 patients, excluding the man who had the shoulder arthrodesis. Three patients complained of significant pain. One was the man with the yet unoperated prosthetic

fracture. A second patient had minimal pain until 18 months after the procedure. At that time,
increasing pain developed and the roentgenographic appearance indicated loosening at the
glenoid bone-cement junction. A third patient
was doing well until 28 months after the procedure. The cause of her recent pain at this time
is uncertain. The remaining eight patients have
only mild pain with use. All eight have had
significant relief of pain and are satisfied in
this respect. Of the 10 patients with intact
prostheses, 4 had no weakness to muscle testing
and 6 had mild weakness. One of the 10 continued
to have tenderness and pain in the area of the
acromioclavicular joint until surgical resection
was accomplished 13 months after the arthroplasty.
One patient, while playing baseball, fractured
his humerus below the prosthesis 22 months after
operation. It has healed readily with plaster
splint immobilization.

14. The averages for active postoperative shoulder motion are shown in Table 2. Evaluation of
functional activities (in the 10 patients with
intact prostheses) indicated that all 10 can use
the operated hand for eating, can dress, can tend
to personal hygiene, and can carry intermediate
weight loads with the extremity. Eight of the 10
can drive an automobile, 8 can sleep on the
operated shoulder, and 7 can comb their hair.
All six of the men can shave. Only four patients
can perform work that requires them to move their
extremity above the shoulder.

15. Roentgenographic evaluation revealed that 10
of the 11 had a radiolucent line at the glenoid
bone-cement junction. This line appeared early,
that is, 3 months after the procedure. It has
not been observed to be of significance during
the follow-up period, except in the one person in
whom pain developed 18 months after operation.
Abduction of the glenohumeral joint as measured
on roentgenograms, with the humeral shaft and the
vertebral border of the scapula used as landmarks,
averaged 18° and ranged from 10° to 28°.

16. As assayed by their responses at the time of
follow-up, two patients had excellent results,
six were satisfied, and three were not improved,
including the one patient with the late fracture
of his prosthesis and the resectional arthroplasty.

DISCUSSION

17. The goal of the operation was to establish a
relatively painless, stable shoulder joint with
enough motion to allow performance of daily
activities. The clinical results indicate that
these goals were not achieved with consistency.
There were immediate problems with the surgical
technique. The limitations in design relative to
function became apparent. With the passage of
time, further shortcomings were noted. Technical
surgical problems with shoulder prosthetic replacement were related to the difficult, often
bloody, exposure. The shoulders that require
total prosthetic replacement commonly have had
trauma or surgery, with resultant scarring and
distortion of the anatomy. Disuse has led to
osteoporosis of skeletal structures, with resulting difficulty in obtaining firm fixation of
prosthetic components. The glenoid fractures
were the result of these hazards.

18. With the 8-mm prosthesis, the head relative
to the high-density polyethylene socket was not
large enough to prevent dislocation, and the 3-mm
neck on the smaller prosthesis was not strong
enough. The need for multiple glenoid placements
at surgery suggested that scapular fixation was
marginal. The two cases of glenoid dislodgements
and the one of loosening illustrate this. The 33°
or 34° of theoretic motion has, in practice, been
approximately 20°. This limited motion represents, in effect, a fibrous ankylosis, with con-
centration of moments at the bond junctions.
This was dramatically illustrated in the man who
had fracture of the humerus at the end of the
stem of the humeral component.

19. We expect further clinical and mechanical
deterioration in these patients. Progressive
loosening of the glenoid components and possibly
fatigue fractures of the neck of the humeral
components may occur. Reoperation in 4 of the 12
patients and the need for revision in 2 (possibly
3) point out that this type of prosthetic shoulder joint replacement is not justified.

20. Currently, we are using a two-part, non-
constrained prosthesis consisting of a chromium-
cobalt humeral component that replaces the humor-
al head and a high-density polyethylene glenoid
dish that resurfaces the articular portion of the
glenoid. Stability is provided by meticulous
immobilization and repair of the capsular-muscle
cuff. This approach has been pioneered by Dr.
Charles S. Neer and the prosthetic design is his.
Our clinical material to date suggests very
satisfactory results: acceptable relief of pain
and active shoulder girdle motion greater than
90° in all planes, with stability. Prosthetic
fracture and loosening have not occurred, and
stability has been achieved without applying
excessive stresses to the implant. Motion is
limited by soft tissues and not by prosthetic
impingement, with the result that stresses are
not transferred to the bone-cement junction.

REFERENCES

1. JONES L. The shoulder joint-observations on
the anatomy and physiology: with an analysis of
a reconstructive operation following extensive
injury. Surg. Gynecol. Obstet. 1942, 75,
October, 433-444.

2. BARR J.S., FREIBERG J.A., COLONNA P.C., and
PEMBERTON P.A. A survey of end results on stabi-
lization of the paralytic shoulder: report of
the Research Committee of the American Orthopaedic
Association. J. Bone Joint Surg. 1942, July,
699-707.

3. BARTON N.J. Arthrodesis of the shoulder for
degenerative conditions. J. Bone Joint Surg.
[Am.] 1972, December, 1759-1764.

4. NEER C.S. II. Displaced proximal humeral
fractures. Part II. Treatment of three-part and
four-part displacement. J. Bone Joint Surg.
[Am.] 1970, 52, September, 1090-1103.

5. NEER C.S. II. Replacement arthroplasty for
glenohumeral osteoarthritis. J. Bone Joint Surg.
[Am.] 1974, 56, January, 1-13.

6. NEER C.S. II. The rheumatoid shoulder. In Surgery of Rheumatoid Arthritis. Edited by R.L. Cruess and N.S. Mitchell. J.B. Lippincott Company, Philadelphia, 1971, p. 117.

7. INMAN V.T., SAUNDERS J.B.deC.M., and ABBOTT L.C. Observations on the function of the shoulder joint. J. Bone Joint Surg. 1944, 26, January, 1-30.

8. REEVES B., JOBBINS B., and FLOWERS M. Biomechanical problems in the development of a total shoulder endoprosthesis (abstract). J. Bone Joint Surg. [Br.] 1972, 54, February, 193.

Table 1

Mechanical tests of Bickel glenohumeral arthroplasty*

Type of test	Head size (mm)	Applied load to to yield (kg)	Applied load to failure (kg)	Moment arm (cm)	Moment to yield (kg-cm)	Moment to failure (kg-cm)	Results
Pullout	10	...	62.5	...	...	...	Pulled out
Lateral bending	8	107.3	165	0.30	32.2	49.5	Neck fracture
Bending dislocation	10	...	97.7	...	...	...	Dislocated
Bending dislocation	10	60	77.3	0.29	171.6	221.1	Neck fracture
Bending dislocation	10	...	155	0.5	...	775	Neck fracture
Bending dislocation	8	123.6	...	2.54	313.9	...	Yielding initiated

*A limited number of prostheses were available for testing. Test values were extremely variable.

Table 2

Averages of active shoulder girdle motion with Bickel glenohumeral arthroplasty*

Motion	Preoperative (degrees)	Postoperative (degrees)	Change (degrees)
Flexion	57 (20 to 130)†	80 (45 to 110)	+23
Extension	19 (0 to 40)	45 (10 to 80)	+26
Abduction	45 (15 to 90)	67 (20 to 110)	+22
Adduction	25 (0 to 65)	30 (15 to 45)	+5
Internal rotation	63 (0 to 90)	81 (40 to 90)	+18
External rotation	10 (-20 to -45)	15 (0 to 35)	+5

*Clinically measured active ranges of shoulder girdle motion. There was approximately 20° increase in flexion, extension, abduction, and internal rotation with no appreciable change in adduction or external rotation.

†Range in parentheses.

Table 3

Complications after Bickel glenohumeral arthroplasty

Complication	No. of pts	Time from surgery (mo)	Comment
Intraoperative			
Glenoid fractures	4	...	Occurred early in series
Dislocation	1	...	Also dislocated postoperatively
Postoperative			
Glenoid dislodgement	2	1/4, 6	Required 1 replacement, 1 arthrodesis
Prosthetic humeral neck fracture	2	8, 38	Involved 8- and 10-mm prostheses, 1 replacement
Dislocation	1	1	Involved 8-mm prosthesis; replaced with 10-mm prosthesis
Loosening	1	18	Increased glenoid bone-methacrylate lytic line and pain
Humerus fracture	1	22	Healed with conservative treatment

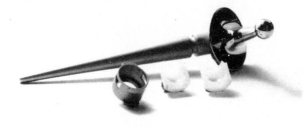 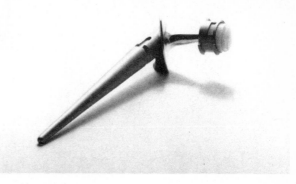

(a) The 10mm humeral component of chromium-cobalt alloy, the two high density polyethylene hemispheres, and the chromium-cobalt enclosing unit

(b) Articulated prosthesis

Fig. 1: Bickel glenohumeral prosthesis

19

20

THE LIVERPOOL TOTAL REPLACEMENT FOR THE GLENO-HUMERAL JOINT

F.H. BEDDOW, MChOrth, FRCS,
Liverpool Royal Infirmary

M.A. ELLOY, PhD, CEng, MIMechE,
S I E Ltd, Southport and BioEngineering Unit, University of Liverpool

SYNOPSIS The gleno-humeral prosthesis utilises a reversed anatomical configuration and provides a natural range of movement together with inherent stability and excellent stem fixation in the axillary border of the scapula. The one size, bilateral prosthesis is self aligning during insertion with protection of the bearing surfaces against accidental damage and ingress of cement. Stability is limited to allow dislocation under traumatic load with prospect of closed reduction. Early results from clinical trials are encouraging.

1. INTRODUCTION

The gleno-humeral is a particularly difficult joint for which to design a satisfactory replacement prosthesis. The normal shoulder enjoys the greatest range of movement of all the major synovial joints. Between full extension and full flexion the arm moves through about 220° and between full internal and full external rotation about 180°. Approximately two thirds of shoulder movement takes place at the gleno-humeral joint. To obtain such a great range of movement the normal shoulder has a very shallow socket which does not significantly encompass the head of the humerus. Stability is achieved mainly by the action of the supraspinatus and the other surrounding muscles although the rather lax capsule and the glenoid with its labrum play a small part. The difficulty of prosthetic design is enhanced by the structure of the scapula which is less than ideal for firm prosthetic fixation.

1.1 Although the need for total replacement of the gleno-humeral joint is found in some cases of bad fracture dislocation, the occasional case of primary osteoarthritis and the rare case of resection of the upper part of the humerus for tumours, the most important indication is in rheumatoid arthritis. Rheumatoid involvement of the shoulder is not rare and the resulting pain and limitation of movement greatly increase the disability arising from multiple involvement of other joints. Unfortunately it is in these rheumatoid joints that the greatest difficulties arise for the design of a satisfactory replacement prosthesis.

2. THE RHEUMATOID SHOULDER

In the rheumatoid shoulder muscular control and stability of the gleno-humeral joint is frequently impaired not only by the gross muscle wasting but also by the complete rupture of the supraspinatus muscle which is impossible to repair. It is therefore felt necessary to enhance the stability of the shoulder by providing a prosthesis with a ball and socket joint having a socket deep enough to provide stability and yet shallow enough to allow an acceptable range of movement.

2.1 The other special problem encountered with the rheumatoid shoulder arises because of the extensive erosion of bone that frequently occurs in the upper and anterior part of the glenoid. This erosion renders the bone in this situation unsuitable for firm prosthetic fixation. However, the axillary border of the scapula is normally intact even in severe rheumatoid disease.

2.2 The axillary border of the scapula is a strong buttress of bone supporting the glenoid. Dissection has demonstrated that it has a medullary cavity about 7 cm long which is capable of accommodating the stem of an intramedullary prothesis.

3. THE ORIGINAL PROSTHESIS

With particular reference to the rheumatoid shoulder the conventional cobalt chrome ball and socket prosthesis, shown in figures 1 and 2, was designed in 1969 and the medullary cavity of the axillary border was used for its scapular fixation. After numerous post mortem insertions, during which it was found that the shape of the stem of the scapular component made it self-aligning within the axillary border, a clinical series of four insertions was made.

3.1 Follow up observation of these patients has shown that no clinical or radiological loosening can be detected after 3 years. Complete pain relief has been achieved and a particularly pleasing observation has been the development of the previously very wasted deltoid muscle indicating that good use is being made of the replaced shoulder.

3.2 The results in this small pilot series were very satisfactory but the design of the prosthesis did not allow full abduction because of impingement of the greater tuberosity on the acromion. There was also insufficient stability to allow early movement before the formation of a new fibrous capsule.

4. DESIGN OBJECTIVE FOR THE NEW PROSTHESIS

Encouraged by this early success it was decided to design a new prosthesis, which utilised this excellent scapular fixation, but also provided the stability and range of movement required. In accordance with the design criteria described by Elloy et al (1) the following design objectives were used:-

4.1 Anatomical centre of articulation - to avoid acromial impingement and to re-establish normal muscle actions.

4.2 Anatomical range of movement - to prevent the prosthesis itself limiting normal active movement and therefore possibly resulting in unacceptable stresses in the implant and its fixation.

4.3 Inherent but limited stability - to compensate for the loss of natural stability and allowing early mobilisation of the joint but capable of dislocation to avoid fracture of the implant or bone under traumatic loads.

4.4 Automatic alignment during insertion - to achieve the design range of movement without the need for special instrumentation.

4.5 Bearing surface protection - to avoid accidental damage to the critical bearing surfaces during surgery and also to avoid the ingress of cement.

4.6 One size with bi-lateral capability - so that the same prosthesis may be used on any shoulder.

5.   THE NEW PROSTHESIS

It was decided that these objectives could best be met by adopting a 'reversed anatomical' configuration similar to that pioneered by Reeves (2) in the 'Leeds Shoulder' which largely met the design objectives but in the opinion of the authors, had the disadvantages of excessive stability, relatively difficult surgery and an over complex design leading to excessive manufacturing cost. The new prosthesis shown in figures 3 and 4 consists of a stainless steel, ball-headed scapular component captively articulating with an ultra-high-molecular-weight-polyethylene humeral cup.

5.1 The scapular component has a 20 mm diameter ball connected by means of a conical neck to the specially shaped cementation stem. A shoulder at the junction of neck and stem, which is normally placed in the plane of the glenoid, facilitates insertion and removal. Correctly inserted, the centre of the ball lies approximately 25 mm from the normal articular surface of the glenoid.

5.2 The humeral component is a 30 mm diameter hemispherical cup suitably grooved on the outside to enhance cemented fixation in the neck of the humerus. The 20 mm diameter, internal, hemispherical form is locally extended by two diametrically opposed 5 mm high lugs, which retain the scapular ball as shown in figure 3. These lugs are reinforced by a metal clip of 3 mm diameter stainless steel wire, which passes over the pole of the cup and bisects the lugs. This clip also acts as an X-ray marker, as shown in figure 7.

5.3 A suitably shaped plastic cap, which snaps onto the neck of the scapular component, as shown in figure 4, complements the humeral cup to completely cover the articulating surfaces and to hold the neck against the equatorial margin of

the cup at a point midway between the two retaining lugs. Rotation about the neck axis produces suitable implantation positions for left or right shoulders and removal of the cap after successful cementation allows a full articulation range.

6. IN VITRO TESTS

6.1 Prosthetic articulation

This is limited by impingement of the neck of the scapular component on the rim of the humeral cup. This permits 145° circumduction over 240° of rotation about the neck axis, but movement is progressively reduced to 85° at the two diametrically opposed points corresponding to the position of the stabilising lugs. It was intended that this reduced articulation should coincide with an arm movement from neutral rotation and full adduction (a position naturally hanging at the side) to maximum abduction without rotation. Figures 5 and 6 show how acromial impingement is avoided in this position. As with the natural joint further arm abduction is achieved by a combination of external rotation, which moves the neck clear of the lugs, and natural scapular movements. Such an implanted position gives no prosthetic limit to flexion/extension and an internal/external rotation range of 145°. Internal rotation is essential for reaching the lumbar spine region. several cadaveric insertions were made to determine the optimum relative orientation of the prosthetic components during insertion and it was found that when the arm was in full adduction and external rotation (i.e. the elbow flexed to 90°, lying by the side of the trunk and with the forearm pointing 10-15° from forward), then the prosthetic components should lie in a position of relative symmetry with the neck of the scapular component resting against the equatorial margin of the humeral cup. This position provides excellent surgical access from an anterior approach and a simple, non-handed design for the complementary cup required to hold the prosthetic components in the correct relative positions during insertion. It was found from cadaveric insertions that in spite of rigor mortis, which must have limited scapular movement, a normal range of arm movement was possible. Impingement of the prosthetic neck on a retaining lug, with a consequent tendency to dislocate, only occurred when the arm was raised about 120° to the body with the palm of the hand facing forward and attempts were made to press the arm backwards, behind the frontal plane - a most uncomfortable position even for a normal healthy joint.

6.2 Stability

The degree of inherent stability required is that which will allow active shoulder movement without the fear of dislocation before natural stability has developed. Reeves (3) has shown that failure of the rotator cuff of the natural joint occurs at about 300-1000 N. The authors considered that an inherent prosthetic stability of only half this would suffice, and also minimise the forces which could be applied to the prosthesis and its fixation. Two cadaveric insertions were made and the articulated prosthesis removed with the scapula and the proximal humerus. Using a 10 kN Howden universal testing machine, the forces to cause prosthetic disarticulation and disruption of prosthetic fixation were measured. To pull the humeral cup off the scapular ball required a force of 140 N directed along the neck axis, and 260 N along the humeral shaft. Disarticulation of the prosthesis at the limits of movement was caused by an external rotation moment of 3.3 Nm and an abduction moment of 0.9 Nm. The lower figure is caused by impingement of the stabilising lugs on the neck of the scapular component. Assuming that these limits of articulation are not reached by the implanted prosthesis an adequate level of stability has been achieved. However, closed reduction, after deliberate dislocation, was achieved in post mortem tests.

6.3 Fixation

The humeral cup fixation was tested by drilling keying holes in the articular surface and cementing a mandrel in position so that the cup was maintained expanded as if a humeral ball was articulated. A pull of 1.11 kN directed along the axis of symmetry caused failure of the bone cement interface. As this was approximately eight times that force which causes disarticulation, cup fixation was considered to be adequate. Attempts to pull the prosthesis out of the scapula, by a force directed parallel to the fixation stem, failed when the scapula broke some distance from the axillary border under a force of 1.57 kN.

The price paid for stability together with a natural centre of articulation is that significant joint forces may be applied to the scapular component at the end of a 25 mm long lever. This imposes moments to this component, tending to twist the scapular stem in its cemented bed. This was considered to be the weakest aspect of the prosthetic fixation so destructive tests were conducted to evaluate it. The weakest load direction corresponded to compressive load along the straight arm when flexed at 90° and adducted 30°. However it is unlikely that significant loads could naturally occur in this direction. Tests were therefore carried out at 90° flexion with neutral adduction, which corresponds to falling onto outstretched arms. Disarticulation of the prosthesis did not occur but at a force of 740 N the axillary border of the scapula cracked with posterior displacement of the prosthetic head. On removal of the load the prosthesis returned to the implanted position with little apparent damage.

7 THE OPERATION

The arthroplasty operation is performed through an anterior approach detaching the anterior one third of the deltoid.

7.1 An oseotomy of the coracoid process is performed and it is displaced downwards on its muscular attachments. The subscapularis is divided and the capsule incised. The head of the humerus is excised through the anatomical neck allowing an excellent view of the glenoid to be obtained. The scapula is then prepared for insertion of the prosthesis by excavating the glenoid with a small gouge and the medullary cavity of the axillary border of the scapula with a small finger reamer. The surgeon's finger passed along the outside of the axillary border of the scapula acts as a useful guide. An excavation is then made in the upper part of the humerus. After a trial insertion the articulated prosthesis is cemented in the scapula and the humerus is reduced onto the humeral component, which is cemented in position with the arm by the side and in 10° - 15° of external rotation. The protective cap is then removed and the range of movement tested.

7.2 Post operatively a closed suction drain is used for about 48 hours. The arm is rested in a sling but, after 4 days, active internal rotation and passive flexion and abduction are encouraged. Active assisted abduction and flexion are commenced after 4 weeks.

8. CLINICAL RESULTS

A clinical evaluation programme is in progress with 9 prostheses implanted between 1975 and 1977. However the time interval is too short to allow final conclusions to be drawn.

8.1 The early results are encouraging. Relief of the severe pre-operative pain is rapid. Internal rotation is achieved easily enabling the patient to reach behind the lumbar spine in about 3 weeks. External rotation to the maximum of 15° beyond neutral is also readily obtained. The wasted and weak deltoid muscle makes it difficult to obtain a full range of active flexion and abduction and at first the movements are best performed with gravity eliminated. The prosthesis allows a full range but preliminary estimates indicate that at present about 120° of active abduction and flexion is being obtained.

REFERENCES

(1) Elloy, M.A., Wright, J.T.M. and Cavendish, M.E. The basic requirements and design criteria for total joint prostheses. Act. Orthorp. Scand. 47, 193-202, 1976.

(2) Reeves, B., Jobbins, B., Dowson, D., and Wright, V. A total shoulder endo-prosthesis Engineering in Medicine V.1, No. 3 64-67. 1972.

(3) Reeves, B. Experiments on the Tensile Strength of the Anterior Capsular Structures of the Shoulder in Man J. Bone Jt. Surg., 50B, 858-865.

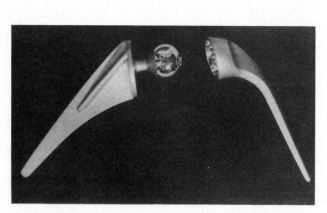

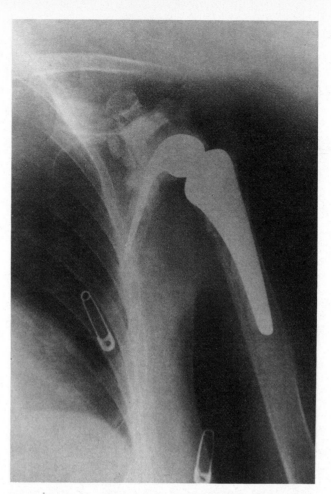

Fig. 1: Original cobalt-chromium total shoulder prosthesis showing humeral component on the left and scapular component on the right

Fig. 2: Original prosthesis implanted showing stemmed scapular fixation in axillary border

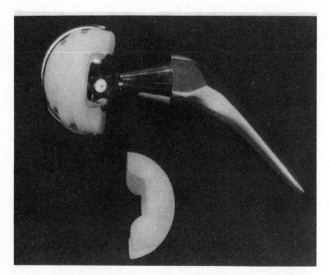

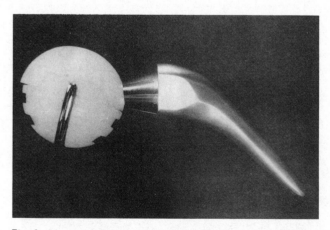

Fig. 3: Liverpool gleno-humeral prosthesis showing prearticulated UHMWP humeral cup with reinforcing clip on left and stainless steel scapular component on right. The complementary plastic cap is shown below

Fig. 4: Liverpool gleno-humeral prosthesis showing protective cap in position

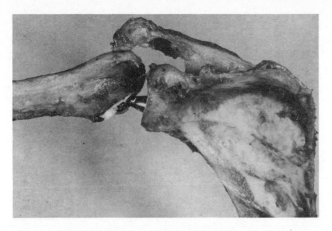

Fig. 5: Cadaveric insertion of the prosthesis showing humerus in full abduction without rotation

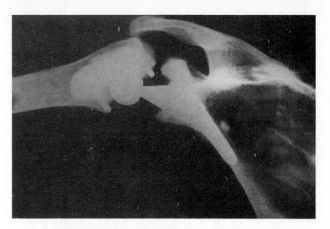

Fig. 6: X-ray of Fig. 5 showing clearance between greater tuberosity and acromion

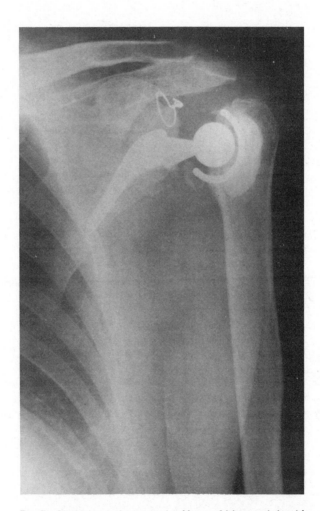

Fig. 7: Clinical anterior-posterior X-ray of Liverpool shoulder in full adduction

C153/77

THE NON-BLOCKED SHOULDER ENDO-PROSTHESIS

A. SIEGEL, H.W.BUCHHOLZ, E. ENGELBRECHT, J. RÖTTGER
Endo-Klinik, Hamburg, West Germany

SYNOPSIS   The results of continous development in prosthetic design of total shoulder joint endoprostheses are a blocked and a non-blocked type of prosthesis. The shoulder joint endo-prosthesis, design 'St.Georg' is a non-blocked system with a head measuring 39 mm in diameter and a polyethylene cup of two different models. Since March 1974 this type of prosthesis has been implanted into 28 shoulder joints with rheumatoid arthritis, ankylosing spondylitis, post-traumatic conditions, arthrosis and tumours as well as in cases with exchange operations where a partial prosthesis was removed and a total prosthesis inserted. The results are satisfactory, since with the prosthesis patients experience relief from pain and improvement of joint movability.

INTRODUCTION

1.   The need for alloarthroplasty of the shoulder joint is not so great as the need for total replacement of the weight-bearing joints of the lower extremities. For many years a partial replacement of the shoulder joint was used in cases of tumours and some particular types of bone fracture. In all these cases only the humeral portion of the joint was replaced, not the glenoid. So far the NEER prosthesis has been a favourite among the many other designs used, but none of all these shoulder joint prostheses was secure against dislocation.

2.   The arthrodesis of the shoulder joint is no alternative for this problem, since here we are faced with residual pain conditions within the region of the cervical muscles which have to carry the arm as well and, furthermore, we encounter technical problems in performing an arthrodesis of the shoulder joint as may be derived from the many various methods prescribed in literature. In addition, strong musculature and stable bones are mandatory in cases of arthrodesis.

Characteristics of shoulder joint prostheses

3.   Different ideas on the construction of a total replacement of the shoulder joint have led to two basicly different types of prostheses. The one is a blocked system, secure against dislocation. A relatively small diameter ball is used as part of the humeral component (5, 7, 10, 11) or the ball is firmly fixed to the glenoid component (4, 8), whereby the ball is held quite firm-ly within the humeral part of the prosthesis by a retention ring. This type of prosthesis gives the shoulder joint a fixed centre of motion and therefore offers a good working point for the power of the deltoid muscle.

But not many experiences have been reported on this blocked system, and the risk factor here is loosening due to catch of both components in cases of severe stress or material breakage.
In other systems the glenoid cavity and the shaft-prosthesis are not joined together (1, 3). Both parts are held in place by the surrounding soft tissues and the rotator cuffs safeguarding both components against dislocation.

Development of shoulder joint endo-prosthesis, design 'St.Georg'

4.   The prosthesis design 'St.Georg' is one of the non-blocked systems. It was developed from a NEER prosthesis combined with an oval polyethylene glenoid cup (STELLBRINK). The results of this system (8 cases from 1971 - 1973) were satisfactory and set impulses to further development.
Cadaveric specimens were measured in order to gain average measurements for a new construction. We took nine measurements from the outside circumference of the humeral head and the glenoid cup and estab-lished the angulation between the head of the humerus and the humeral shaft as well as the angle of retrotorsion of the humeral head to the axis of the elbow joint (STELLBRINK). The measurements significant for the construction of a shoulder joint endo-prosthesis are shown in (Fig. 1).

Characteristics of the shoulder joint endo-prosthesis, design 'St.Georg' (Fig. 2)

5.   The design being in use since March 1974 has a humeral head prosthesis fabri-cated of cobalt-chromium-molybdenum alloy with a 39 mm Ø head. The head with a

polished surface is larger than a hemispherical ball and joined with a tapering stem at a 45° angle of inclination. The total length of the prosthetic stem from the centre of the head to its end is 100 mm. On the tubercular side of the prosthesis shaft and head form a continuous line while on the joint aspect of the prosthesis the head overlaps. The shaft is grooved to secure a firm fixation to the humerus.
In case there is need for replacement of larger portions of the proximal humeral bone we have a special prosthesis available with a longer stem surrounded with a polyethylene cuff in length of bone resection. In two cases we have chosen a special total metal construction instead of using a polyethylene cuff (9). In another case we replaced the total humerus together with the implantation of a total shoulder and elbow joint prosthesis, design 'St.Georg'.
The glenoid cup is replaced by a polyethylene model embracing the polished humeral head by approximately 1/4 (one quarter) of its circumference. According to anatomical conditions two different cup models are used:
1) a circular glenoid cup with a diameter of 35 mm and a measured depth of 10 mm. The cup has a pivot at the back and a relief surface finish to provide firm fixation in bone cement;
2) a glenoid cup equipped with a cranial roof is used in any case where due to pathological changes on the humeral bone dislocation towards cranial is very likely to occur due to tensile forces of the muscles. Since a displacement of the humeral head towards cranial involves displacement of the turning point within the shoulder joint with following dislocation this may be prevented by the roof on the upper rim of the glenoid cup. This special cup provides secure abutment for the humeral head on active abduction of the arm.
The prosthesis can be used for either the right or the left shoulder. Both components of the shoulder joint endo-prosthesis are cemented into place with Refobacin-Palacos^R

Operative technique

6.   The operation is performed with the patient supine and the joint placed on an armtable. The affected shoulder is slightly elevated. A S-shaped skin incision is applied from the acromion along the ventral margin of the musculus deltoides to the lateral side of the humerus. The deltoid muscle is divided by blunt dissection in its ventral portion, so that only in cases with an overly developed musculature parts of the pars clavicularis must be mobilized. The long biceps tendon is divided above the attachment of the musculus pectoralis major and mobilized from its tendinous canal to its site of insertion at the upper margin of the glenoid cup.
The rotator cuffs of the subscapularis muscle the supraspinatus and the infraspinatus together with a musculus teres minor are successively exposed and then detached from their insertion by sharp incision. After retraction of the joint capsule from the medial portion of the humeral shaft the head is easily dislocated.

7.   After resecting the head of the humerus down to the collum anatonicum we have a free view on the glenoid cup. In cases of rheumatoid arthritis we now perform a total synovectomy. The joint capsule is preserved, as within the capsule there are the deep fibres of the rotator cuff attachments, detached from the humeral bone. The cup is centrally reamed with a special reamer. The shape of the cup corresponds to the back part of the polyethylene cup. The central drill hole is undermined and in addition, special fixation holes are drilled. The head prosthesis is inserted in approximately 20° retrotorsion. Head and cup are cemented in place with Refobacin-Palacos^R. During a test run the surgeon has to make sure that there is free play between the acromion and the tubercular region. The mobilized muscle groups are re-attached to their places of origin by means of strong plastic threads guided through the drill holes within the tubercular region. The long biceps tendon is reunited by a Bunnell suture or fixed to the humerus. After wound drainage the deltoid muscle is adapted with single stitches and the skin is closed with monophile plastic thread.

Post-operative management

8.   After the operation the arm is placed on a plastic abduction splint. The splint is of very low weight, can be applied easily and prevents the arm from dorsal displacement while the patient is lying in a supine position. Normally the splint is left on for 4-6 weeks. Active exercises on the wrist and the elbow and also isometric exercises are initiated immediately postoperative. Gentle passive exercises on the shoulder joint are instituted in the second postoperative week. In the third week the splint may be removed temporarily for pendulum exercises. Active exercises may start after the fourth postoperative week and be gradually increased.

Indications

9.   Since March 1974 28 patients have received a total shoulder joint endo-prosthesis, design 'St.Georg'. Rheumatoid arthritis occupied 1/3 (one third) of the indications for the prosthesis. The next following group involved patients with post-traumatic conditions (arthrosis, headnecrosis, old crushing fractures). The rest of the patients had arthrosis, tumours, or a partial shoulder joint prosthesis without cup replacement. One patient had a remobilized arthrodesis of the shoulder joint.
22 patients were female (average age 57 years and a half; 29 - 77 years).
6 patients were male (average age 59 years and a half; 44 - 76 years).

Results

10.   Our follow-up investigations on 24 patients operated on until the end of 1975 have shown that patients with rheumatoid arthritis had obtained the best results. To these patients relief from pain and maintenance of joint movability or even improve-

ment of functional movement is of great significance. Patients with post-traumatic conditions were in some cases left with tolerable residual pains. In 2 cases of post-traumatic arthrosis with paresis of the nervus axillaris due to an accident the results were unsatisfactory. In one of these cases we had an arthrodesis of the shoulder joint remobilized.

In one case with syringomyelia we observed late infection and, considering the basic disease, removed the prosthesis. Out of 3 patients with tumours 2 had metastases. Meanwhile these patients have died. The implantation of a shoulder joint endo-prosthesis has given these patients immediate relief from pain. The third patient, a female, suffered from primary tumor within the proximal portion of the humeral bone. She is now able to work. Her joint movability is satisfactory. She experienced dislocation of the joint towards cranial as nothing of the rotator cuffs was left. Re-operation was ommitted since the patient was satisfactory with her result.

In one patient with rheumatoid arthritis we exchanged the cup due to cranial dislocation. Poor joint movability and pain conditions due to cranial displacement of the turning point were significantly improved after exchange of the circular cup to a cup with a cranial roof.

From our own observations we know that on the average patients improved their joint movability between 20 and 60 degrees abduction and elevation.

Evaluation

11.   The use of a non-blocked type of shoulder prosthesis according to the low friction principle enables us to eliminate pain from the severely damaged shoulder joint with maintenance of stability or even functional improvement of the joint.
A review on 28 replacement operations of the shoulder joint with the design 'St.Georg' together with the evaluation of 8 shoulder joint prostheses inserted by STELLBRINK show that total replacement of the joint outweighs the previous replacements of only the humeral portion of the joint. The initially feared risk of dislocation in an un-blocked system has not proven entirely true. Only in cases of inefficient soft tissues, weak rotator cuffs or even nerve deficiencies we must anticipate dislocation. In non-blocked designs wandering of the turning point within the shoulder joint may occur according to physiological conditions. Luxation will only occur when severe stress is applied to the joint, as it would happen in normal joints also.
In order to guarantee free abduction we need a secure abutment for the humeral head against the shoulder blade. In the early phase of abduction we need a secure cranial support. If the anatomical conditions are unsatisfactory in this respect abutment is provided with the earlier described roof on the upper rim of the glenoid cup.

Discussion

12.   Delimitation of indications for the shoulder joint endo-prosthesis to alternate procedures is not a subject to be discussed here, longer periods of observation are needed.
Discussions on the question, whether a blocked shoulder joint endo-prosthesis and consequently a fixed turning point is acceptable or whether those prostheses guided by the surrounding soft tissues will have the better long-term results will continue for years.
The preliminary results of both systems seem to show no significant differences, though unfortunately we have observed fractures of material. We are of the opinion that two non-blocked prosthetic components guided by the surrounding soft tissues are as near anatomy as possible.
The question regarding the material most suited for fabricating the prosthesis may be solved analogous to the evaluation of materials for hip joint replacement.

REFERENCES

1.   CAFFINIERE J.Y. Prothese totale d'epaule. Editions Inserm, Paris, 1975

2.   ENGELBRECHT E. und STELLBRINK G. Total shoulder replacement, design 'St.Georg'. Scand J.Rheumatology 4:suppl 8,1975.

3.   ENGELBRECHT E. und STELLBRINK G. Totale Schulterendoprothese Modell "St.Georg". Chirurg 1976 - im Druck.

4.   KÖLBEL R. und FRIEDEBOLD Schulterprothese nach Kölbel-Friedebold. 6.Reisensburger Workshop 2.-4.Sept.1976 - im Druck Verlag Hans Huber, Bern.

5.   LETTIN A.W.F. and SCALES J.T. Total replacement of the shoulder joint. Proc.Royal Soc.65,373-374(1972).

6.   NEER C.S. The rheumatoid shoulder. In surgery of rheumatoid arthritis. Philadelphia-Toronto J.B. Lippincott 1972.

7.   POST M. and HASKELL S. Total shoulder replacement. Orth.rev.IV,53-57(1975).

8.   REEVES B. et al. A total shoulder endo-prosthesis. Engineering in Medicine 1, 64-67(1972)

9.   SIEGEL A., ENGELBRECHT E. und RÖTTGER J. Teilersatz des Oberarmknochens. Chir.47 im Druck (1976).

10. WEIGERT M. und GRONERT H.-J. Totaler Schultergelenksersatz. Zbl.Chir.100, 1037-1044(1975).

11. ZIPPEL J. Arthroplastik des Schultergelenkes. Orth.,2,107-109(1973).

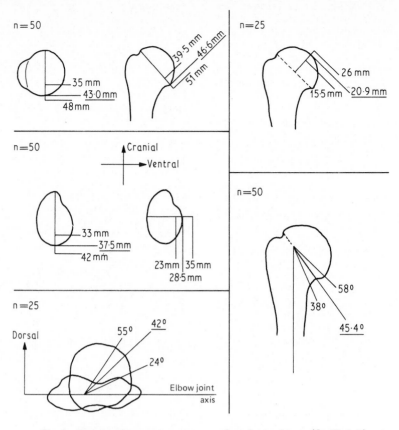

Fig. 1: Results of measurements on cadaveric specimens (Stellbrink)

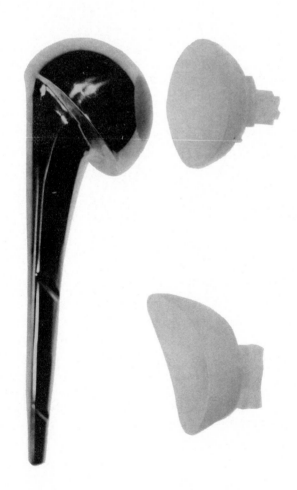

Fig. 2: Total shoulder endo-prosthesis, design 'St. Georg'

30

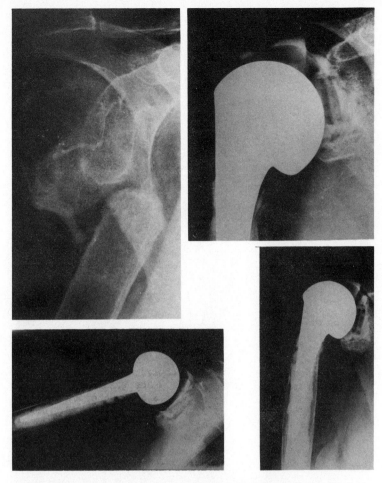

Fig. 3: Female, 76 years, pseudarthrosis of the humerus after several
operations and appearance 1 year after the operation

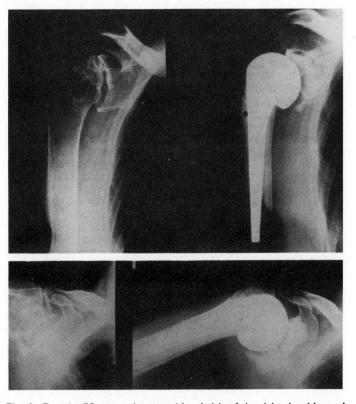

Fig. 4: Female, 52 years, rheumatoid arthritis of the right shoulder and
the lower arm one year after the operation

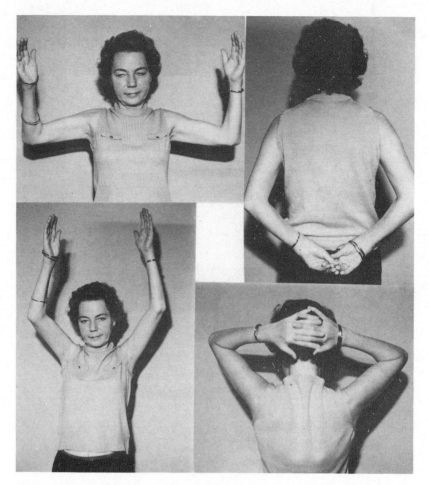

Fig. 5: The same patient, clinical result one year after the operation

C154/77

ARTHROPLASTY OF THE UPPER LIMB. LINK ARTHROPLASTY OF THE ELBOW. LINK ARTHROPLASTY OF THE METACARPO-PHALANGEAL JOINTS — A PROGRESS REPORT

M.B. DEVAS, MChir, FRCS, and V. SHAH, FRCS
Royal East Sussex Hospital, Hastings

SYNOPSIS   In this paper link arthroplasty of the elbow is described and a follow-up of link arthroplasty of the metacarpo-phalangeal joints is given.

THE ELBOW

1.   The principle of link arthroplasty has already been described both for the knee and for the finger (Devas 1974) (Ref. 1); (Devas 1974), (Ref. 2); (Devas and Shah 1975)   (Ref. 3), and it is not proposed to describe in detail how the link prosthesis locks into itself.   However, it is important to recall that, because of the simple nature of a male component locking into a female component there is no need to remove an excessive amount of bone, and only a small part of the joint is removed into which the two components are placed.   Therefore, if salvage is necessary, bone length has not been lost.   In the elbow the normal method of linking the prosthesis is reversed.   The humeral component has a high density polythene articulation shaped like a cotton reel, similar to the normal trochlea, and the ulnar component of Vinertia locks on to this.   Because the ulnar component is just over half a circle in shape, there has to be the usual notch in the humeral component to allow the prostheses to lock together in full flexion.   The humeral component occupies the position of the lateral part of the trochlea, with the stem up the humeral shaft.   The ulnar stem fits into a hole reamed down the ulna but also the joint surface of the olecranon has to be removed (in rheumatoid arthritis it has usually been destroyed) to accommodate the prosthesis which replaces it completely. Figure 1 shows the prosthesis.

The technique of operation.

2.   The elbow is approached through a curved lateral incision which starts anteriorly in the midline above the elbow, curving laterally round the epicondyle and ending up toward the midline in the upper forearm.   The skin and sub- cutaneous tissues are reflected medially both anteriorly and posteriorly and the ulnar nerve identified.

3.   The head of the radius is usually removed before cutting through the olecranon at the distal joint level. The olecranon process is reflected posteriorly.   A drill hole is then made upwards from the centre of the trochlea into the humeral shaft.   This is because if it is left until after the central part of the trochlea has had the notch cut out of it to accommodate the humeral part of the prosthesis it can be difficult to enter the humeral shaft through the very thin bone adjacent to the olecranon fossa.   Sufficient width of the trochlea is removed, the hole up the shaft of the humerus enlarged by a hand reamer and the humeral component is given a trial fit.   If this is satisfactory, the ulna shaft is then reamed out; it is important not to use a power tool because, especially in rheumatoid arthritis, it is easy to broach the ulna cortex.   At the same time the joint surface of the olecranon is deepened.   If the trial fit is satisfactory then the two components are cemented in and the joint locked together.

4.   Just before the ulnar component is pushed home a wire is passed through a small hole at the base of the stem which is used to wire the olecranon back into its normal position.   The wound is closed and a pressure bandage applied in the usual way.

Programme after operation

5.   Early gentle movements are allowed. The pressure bandage is removed at two days with the suction drains.   Gradually the arm is allowed increasing movements.

Results.

6.   The initial results were good but loosening of the prosthesis is a serious problem.

Table 1

Material

Number of patients:	9
Men:	3
Women:	6
Diagnosis:	Rheumatoid arthritis

33

Table 2

RESULTS

Outcome in months

Case number	Satisfactory	Loose
1	34	
2	30	
3	41	
4		48
5	43	
6		19
7		3 (infected)
8		6 (replaced)
9	20	

Discussion.

7.   Link arthroplasty of the elbow is a simple procedure that leaves most of the natural elbow joint present, including the capsule and ligaments. It is a metal-to-plastic prosthesis but the long term results do not warrant continuing this method at the moment, because of loosening.   It is thought that this is because there is no provision for joint distraction.   Unlike the knee joint in which link arthroplasties have remained satisfactory for many years, the elbow suffers a great deal more distraction in certain movements and in rheumatoid arthritis the lax ligaments do not protect the joint from stretching.   Nevertheless, because the principle of the operation removes so little bone it has been found possible to salvage these joints by using the stabilised gliding elbow prosthesis (Attenborough 1976) (Ref. 4)

8.   It is a consolation that despite the early good results, not many cases were done.   This should always be the case with a new prosthesis or technique.   Failure to observe a few early results for a long time can lead to a disaster from the wholesale implanting of a new prosthesis.

Case 1.

9.   A girl of twenty-five had had juvenile rheumatoid arthritis which continued into adult life.   She was a school teacher and complained that she could not hold the chalk because her left thumb gave way. In August 1970 a link arthroplasty was done on the metacarpo-phalangeal joint of the left thumb.   Three years later she had severe pain in the right elbow (Figure 2) with considerable disability and a link arthroplasty was done in January 1974 (Figures 3 to 5).   In February 1974 a further link arthroplasty was done on the third metacarpo-phalangeal joint of the left hand (Figure 6) because of rheumatoid destruction progress.   The result in the elbow has continued to be satisfactory with a range of flexion from 55 degrees to 150 degrees with 45 degrees of pronation and 20 degrees of supination.

Case 2

10.   A woman of eighty with rheumatoid arthritis had a painful, disorganised right elbow which was replaced in May 1974.   The elbow has remained satisfactory except for a cementoma (Caused by cement leaking out of a hole in the humeral cortex) which has caused some pain but insufficient to make the patient agree to have it removed.

Case 3

11.   A woman of forty-two with rheumatoid arthritis had a painful disorganised left elbow.   In May 1973 this was replaced by a link prosthesis.   Progress was satisfactory after the operation except that movement was poor.   The range of flexion was from 60 degrees to 110 degrees with rotation of 90 degrees.   Apart from this the elbow is satisfactory.

Case 4

12.   A man of sixty-one with severe rheumatoid arthritis had his right elbow replaced in July 1972.   After this, in the same year he had link arthroplasties of the index and middle metacarpo-phalangeal joints of the right hand and in 1974 he had further link arthroplasties of the index, middle and ring fingers of the opposite hand.   The elbow responded well and he was able to flex the elbow from 30 degrees to 110 degrees.   Early in 1976 he started to get pain in the elbow.   There was evidence of loosening and he is awaiting replacement with the stabilised gliding elbow prosthesis.

Case 5

13.   A woman of sixty-three with rheumatoid arthritis had link arthroplasties of the right middle and index metacarpo-phalangeal joints in May 1970 and excision of the head of the right radius at the same time.   Three years later, in February 1973, she had a link arthroplasty of the right elbow.   She regained a range of flexion from 20 to 100 degrees.   She was extremely pleased to be able to get her fingers to her mouth.   The prosthesis has remained satisfactory.

Case 6

14.   A woman of fifty-seven with rheumatoid arthritis had link arthro-plasties of the index and middle metacarpo-phalangeal joints of the right hand.   Four months later in November 1973 she had a link arthroplasty of the right elbow with excision of the radial head.   In March 1975 she had a stabilised gliding knee replacement. The patient developed pain in the elbow early in 1976 and the prosthesis had become loose.   There was a history of a fall which was probably not contributory to the loosening but which may have caused a fracture of the medial

epicondyle. The latter was treated conservatively with reasonable improvement but the prosthesis may well have to be replaced in the future. When last seen the fracture had united and she had a useful range of movement but there was still much aching in the elbow.

Case 7

15. A woman with rheumatoid arthritis had a right link arthroplasty of the elbow in May 1976. She was discharged home six days after the operation as was usual but later developed a discharge containing Staphylococcus albus. This was treated with antibiotics and the wound healed. Three months later a collection of pus had to be evacuated from the elbow and at that time the prosthesis was found to be loose.

Case 8

16. A man of sixty-eight with rheumatoid arthritis had a right elbow replacement in November 1975. He remained extremely well for a few months but, after jerking his arm, began to develop pain. In May 1976 it was obvious that the prosthesis was loose and in August 1976 the link prosthesis was removed and a stabilised gliding elbow prosthesis inserted (Attenborough 1976) (Ref. 5).

Case 9

17. A man of forty-two had a link arthroplasty of the left elbow done in January 1975. The wire that was used to hold the olecranon in place caused some irritation and was removed in January 1976. In May 1976 he complained of an occasional click in the left elbow but he had no severe symptoms. He had a range of movement of 40 degrees to 120 degrees and this elbow is suspect but not proven to be loose at the moment.

THE METACARPO-PHALANGEAL JOINTS.

18. A preliminary report of link arthroplasty of the metacarpo-phalangeal joint was given by Devas and Shah in 1975. The follow-up, completed in 1974, ranged from three months to forty-four months. In this review the average follow-up is four years.

19. In the paper mentioned above it was shown that it was possible to inject cement into the metacarpal and phalangeal shafts so as to obtain a very firm fixation of the two components of the link arthroplasty. Firm fixation has probably caused a worsening of results. When link arthroplasties were first done several patients had the prosthesis inserted without the use of cement and, although it is obvious that each of the latter is loose, the patients still have reasonable results after five years.

20. Because many of the patients chosen for the operation were elderly and suffering from rheumatoid arthritis, many

patients have died since the last follow-up, so that of a total of thirty-three patients with seventy-one metacarpo-phalangeal joints of the fingers operated upon from 1970 to 1974, six patients with fifteen joints have been excluded from the present review because of death and two patients with five joints who failed to attend for review. This left a total of twenty-five patients with fifty-one joints for review, after including patients operated upon since the previous review.

21. There were four males and twenty-one females. The youngest was twenty-four years old and the oldest was eighty-three years old. The average age was sixty-three years. Table 3 shows the number of arthroplasties of the metacarpo-phalangeal joints and this is very similar to that previously recorded.

Table 3

NUMBER OF METACARPO-PHALANGEAL JOINTS	
Index finger	24
Middle finger	24
Ring	2
Little	1
	51

22. Table 4 shows the distribution of the link arthroplasties in the hands and Table 5 the follow-up period.

Table 4

NUMBER OF HANDS	
Index only	2
Middle only	2
Little only	1
Index and middle	20
Index, middle and ring	2

Table 5

FOLLOW UP PERIOD	
Shortest	2 years
Average	4 years
Longest	6 years

23. The results were graded in exactly the same way as previously (Table 6) and the results are shown in Table 7.

Table 6

GRADING OF RESULTS: CRITERIA		
Good	Fair	Bad
Loss of pain	Occasional pain	Pain persistent
Active range of 40° from 20° to 60°	Active range less than in 'good'	Useless finger
Stable joint	Patient satisfied Stable joint	

Table 7

RESULTS

	Number of joints	Percentage
Good	26	50
Fair	10	20
Bad	15	30

Table 8

COMPLICATIONS

Infection	2 (2 patients)
Unusual reaction	2 (1 patient)
Locking	1
Breakage	4

Discussion

24. A total of seventy-one metacarpo-phalangeal joints of fingers were operated upon. Twenty joints were excluded from the review because of intervening death of the patient or failure to attend.

25. Table 7 shows thirty per-cent of the results were bad. This is far too big a figure to make the method freely acceptable. Failure was caused by sepsis, and perhaps a form of sensitivity or reaction to hot cement. In one diabetic rheumatoid patient one joint out of two replaced became infected. In one patient with rheumatoid arthritis eight months after operation ulceration developed over the knuckles of the joints which gradually deepened, necessitating removal of the prosthesis. Extensive invest-igations did not show any cause. It was thought to be necrotic arteritis; alternatively it is possible that necrosis occurred with the metacarpal bone because of the heat engendered by the cement*

26. The main cause of failure in the remainder was caused by loosening of the prosthesis with disruption. This may well have been caused, paradoxically, by better fixation of the prosthetic compon-ents by injecting cement right down the metacarpal and phalangeal shafts. Perhaps less satisfactory fixation allowed some inadvertent pistoning of the prosthesis in the phalanx.

27. The breakages of the metacarpal component were caused by welding failures and have been corrected.

28. Table 7 shows 50 per cent with good results and 20 per cent with fair results. Overall 70 per cent were satisfactory to the patient

* Since the review another patient has had the same complication.

29. For patients with rheumatoid arthritis the improvement in function of the hand by improving the metacarpo-phalangeal joints, especially of the index and middle fingers, can be great, even though in some patients the actual range of flexion decreased. This is because the joint before operation was unstable, with no power to grip.

30. Most arthroplasties with good or fair results showed that the prosthesis in the proximal phalanx had become loose but with no symptoms. With the absolute fixation later in the series, stiffness of the arthroplasty was common or, if loosening occurred, there was disruption.

31. The results, though not good, should be compared to other series of arthroplasties, such as Beckenbaugh, Dobyns, Linscheid and Bryan (1976) (Ref.6)

32. In the light of the findings it is reasonable to suppose that, if the complications and problems of fixation could be overcome, the method might well be given further trial. Good results could be very good (Figures 8 and 9). To this end a modified prosthesis with a different technique of insertion is being considered and will be introduced in due course.

REFERENCES

1. Devas, M. Link Arthroplasty of the Knee in the Knee Joint. Proceedings of the International Congress, Rotterdam, September 13th - 15th 1973. Excerpta Medica, Amsterdam, (1974) Page 248 - 250.

2. Devas, M. Link Arthroplasty of the Knee in Total Knee Replacement. The Institution of Mechanical Engineers, London (1974) 96 - 101.

3. Devas, M. and Shah, V. Link Arthroplasty of the Metacarpo-phalangeal joints. A Preliminary Report of a New Method. The Journal of Bone and Joint Surgery (1975) Vol. 57-B No. 1, pages 72 - 77.

4. Attenborough, 1976 q.v.

5. Attenborough, 1976 q.v.

6. Beckenbaugh, R., Dobyns, J., Linscheid, R. and Bryan, R., Review and Analysis of Silicone Rubber Metacarpo-phalangeal Implants. Journal of Bone and Joint Surgery (1976), 58 A/4 June 1976, pages 483 - 487.

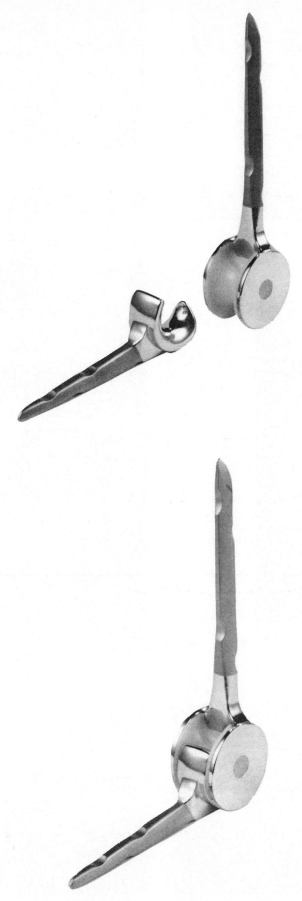

Fig. 1: The link elbow is shown separated. The humeral component is made of Vinertia but with a high density polythene articulation to receive the ulna portion. The notch on the humeral high density polythene insert is seen adjacent to the stem. The prosthesis is also shown assembled. There is no metal to metal contact

37

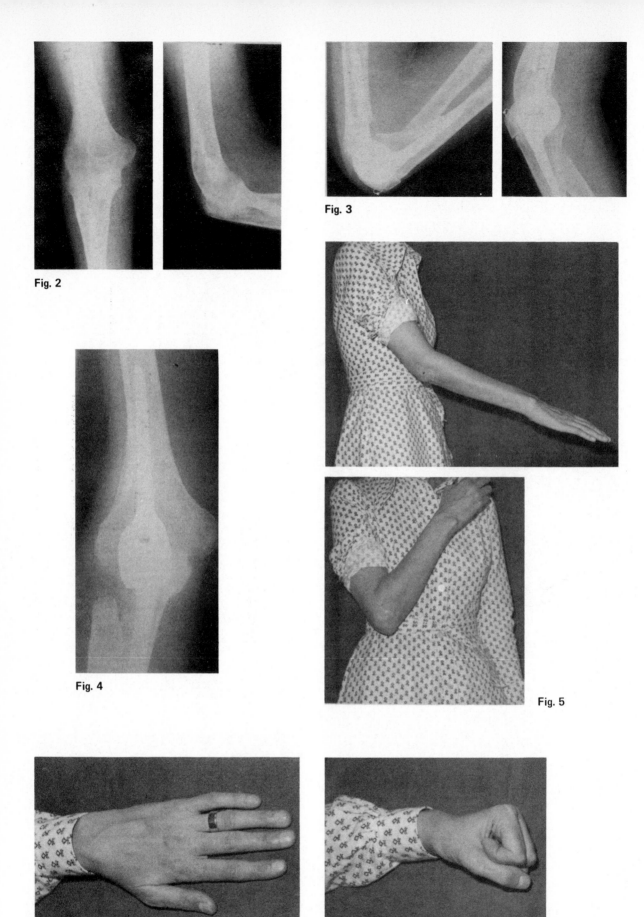

Figs. 2 — 6: Case 1. Figure 2 shows the radiographs of the elbow severely affected by rheumatoid arthritis.
Figure 3 shows lateral radiographs some months after operation to show the range of flexion,
and in Fig. 4 the anteroposterior view (this prosthesis was metal-to-metal). Fig. 5 shows the
clinical appearance. This operation was done through a posterior transverse incision.
Fig. 6 shows the clinical appearance and range of movement of the metacarpo-phalangeal joint
of the left middle finger some months after link arthroplasty

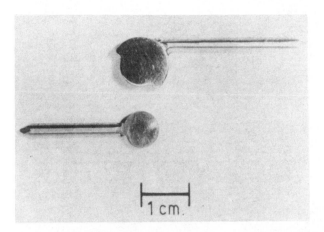 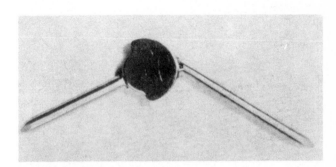

Fig. 7: The link metacarpo-phalangeal joint prosthesis. With the two components separated the notch in the head of the phalangeal portion can be seen adjacent to the base of the stem

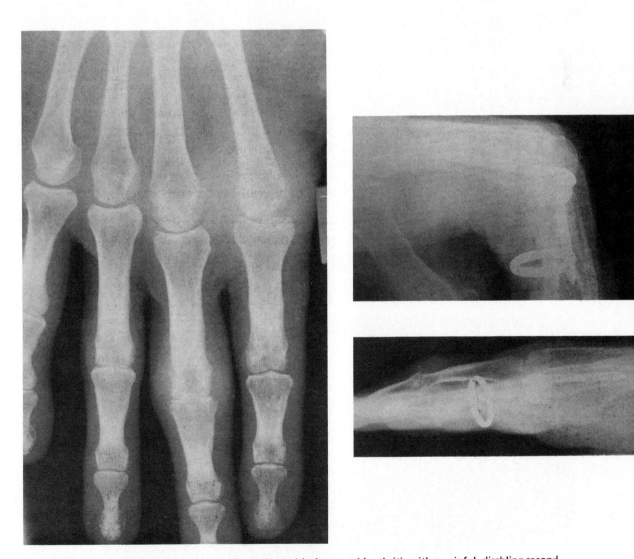

Fig. 8: shows the radiographic appearance of a patient with rheumatoid arthritis with a painful, disabling second metacarpo-phalangeal joint of the index finger before operation and the appearance and range of movement after link arthroplasty

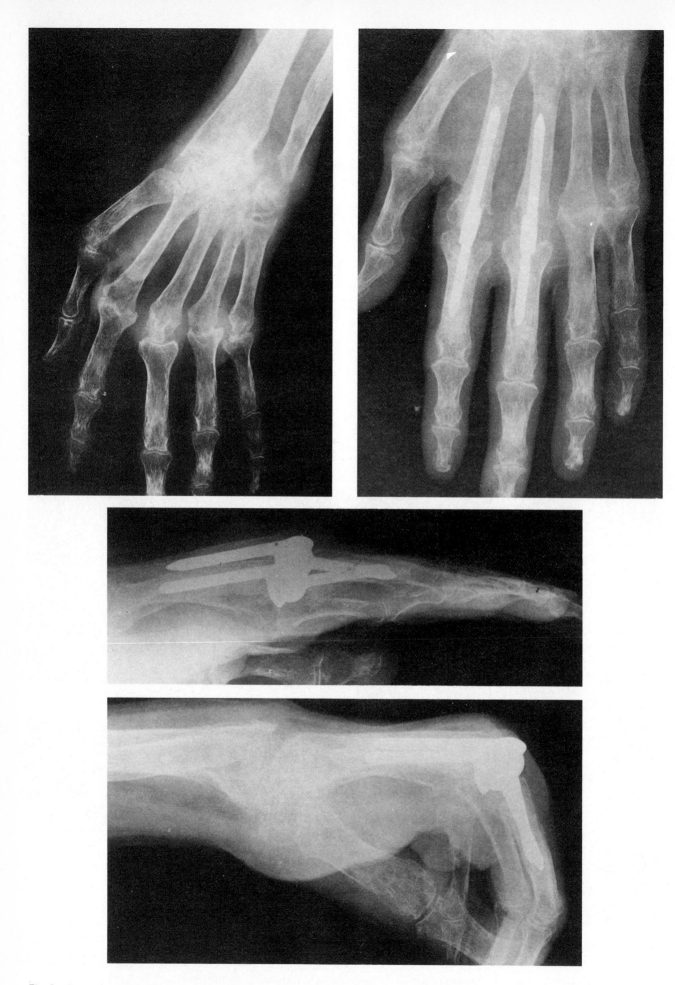

Fig. 9: shows the radiographs of a patient with rheumatoid arthritis before operation and after operation, in which the range of movement is also shown

40

THE OPTIMISED USE OF PMMA BONE CEMENT AND SOME LIMITATIONS OF ITS USE IN THE FIXATION OF UPPER LIMB PROSTHESES

A.J.C. LEE, BSc, PhD, Department of Engineering Science,
University of Exeter, Exeter

R.S.M. LING, FRCS, Princess Elizabeth Orthopaedic Hospital,
Wonford Road, Exeter

SYNOPSIS   The role of PMMA bone cement as a prosthetic fixation medium in the upper limb has been considered. The method of fixation provided by PMMA is described with reference to its successful use in the lower limb. Some failures of fixation are described and conclusions drawn as to the likely success of PMMA in the upper limb.

INTRODUCTION

1.   Acrylic bone cement has now been in use for a great many years and has been remarkably successful in the fixation of implants in the lower limb, particularly at the hip. It has been so successful in fact, that similar success has been expected by many when it is used for the fixation of implants in the upper limb. Developments in the use of artificial joints in the upper limb have been taking place at such a rate that it can do no harm to review briefly the way in which acrylic cement achieves implant fixation. The review can then be used as a basis to assess what can be expected from its use in the upper limb, and thus, by inference, what is unreasonable and therefore perhaps should not be attempted.

Fixation with acrylic cement

2.   Acrylic cement has no adhesive properties whatsoever and achieves fixation basically by mechanical interlocking with host and prosthetic components. This mechanical interlock is usually much as in a jigsaw puzzle, though in addition, the principle of the engineering taper is employed in certain circumstances for the fixation of intramedullary components.

Effect of movement of cement within bone

3.   A point of fundamental importance in the use of acrylic, especially in the upper limb, is an appreciation of the fact that, once acrylic cement starts to move repetitively against or within bone, bone is destroyed, the precise mechanism of this continuing destruction being uncertain. This phenomenon was described originally by McKee and Watson-Farrar in their now classic paper published in 1966, (Ref. 1) and has again been referred to recently in the Journal of Bone and Joint Surgery by Harris and his colleagues from Boston (Ref. 2). The dominant histological feature in the tissue adjacent to the cement in the cases described by Harris was a very marked accumulation of macrophages. An extreme example of this phenomenon at the hip is shewn in figure 1, which shews the hips of a 72 year old man virtually confined to a wheelchair by his osteoarthritis. In 1965 he underwent bilateral total hip arthroplasty and was restored virtually to normal activity for his age. Seven years later, after a fall on board ship, he complained of pain in his knee and eventually, it was appreciated that this pain was arising in the hip. The X-ray appear-

ances are seen in figure 2. The marked bone destruction with apparent cyst formation initially lead to suspicions of infection, but exploration with subsequent bacteriological investigations did not confirm this. A finding of great importance in the interpretation of these X-ray appearances related to the cement just below the lower end of the stem, where there was a plug of cement absolutely firmly fixed in the medullary canal. There was no bone destruction whatsoever at this site; if anything, the reverse. The tip of the stem was resting on this plug, rather like the point of a spinning top, and the stem itself was able to rotate axially, standing on its tip. The cement mass surrounding the distal two thirds of the stem was still attached to the stem and as the stem rotated, this cement mass moved with it, with the consequences seen in the figure. The only site at which cement was not moving against or within bone was at the tip where the plug was firmly fixed, and this area showed no adjacent destruction of bone whatsoever.

4.   This phenomenon of bone destruction due to repetitive movement of acrylic leads to a number of recommendations with regard to implant fixation using acrylic:
i)   The initial implantation of the cement and securing of the cement-bone junction must be meticulous. The area of the cement bone junction should be as large as possible in any given site.
ii)   The loads at the cement bone junction, especially in shear, should be minimised.
iii) If movement at the cement bone junction does start, especially with an intramedullary stem, the configuration and loading pattern should be such as to allow spontaneous tightening under load rather than repetitive movement and thus further destruction of bone, with gross loosening.

Achievement of implant fixation : general

5.   The recommendations must now be considered in turn.
i) The initial implantation of the cement and the securing of the cement-bone junction:
a) The preparation of the bone surface of cavity:
In order for satisfactory mechanical interlocking with host bone to be achieved, the aim should be to apply the cement dough to a clean surface of well supported cancellous bone of 'good' quality. The importance of mechanical cleansing of the bone

surface prior to implantation has been shewn by the work of Miller, (Ref. 3) of Montreal, amongst others, and apart from mechanical cleansing, the use of some type of bone washer to clear the cancellous spaces of fat, debris and blood is advisable. Acrylic cement cannot 'get a grip' on a smooth bone surface, such as is often left following the use of oscillating saws or rotating reamers. The development of fixation pits is necessary on such surfaces; such pits should not have sharp edges which may act as unacceptable stress raisers on the brittle acrylic cement.

b) The application of cement to the bone surface or cavity:
The aim is to force the cement against and into the boney walls of the cavity or surface, and to fill the cavity fully with cement, whilst excluding, in so far as this is possible, blood and tissue debris. Whilst conventional techniques of 'thumbing' cement into the medullary canal of the femur may result in reasonably effective filling, in the upper limb, the much smaller medullary canals and restricted access demand a more refined technique; and the use of a syringe of some type, preferably with retrograde filling, is madatory if efficient filling is to be achieved. Retrograde filling is made more effective with preliminary distal occlusion of the lumen of the canal, though this is perhaps impractical in the upper limb with the exception of the humerus. Added and important advantages of the use of a syringe are, first the complete exclusion of blood from the cement, and second, the fact that pressure is applied to the cement as it is extruded from the syringe. These measures both add to the mechanical strength of the finally cured resin. The latter can be improved further, and extrusion of the cement into the bone surface enhanced by applying further pressure to the cement before polymerisation. This entails the presence or creation of a closed cavity to allow, by various techniques, the development of increased pressure on the cement. The introduction of a tapering intramedullary stem has this effect; a parallel sided stem is less effective and carries with it the risk of the creation of voids between the stem and the cement if the stem is moved at all out of alignment within the medullary canal before polymerisation.

ii) The loads at the cement bone junction, especially in shear, should be minimised:

This has implications for the materials and geometry of the artificial joint components. Under load, the bearing surfaces of the joint must generate minimal frictional forces, because such forces will be transmitted straight to the cement bone junction in the form of shear. Thus a metal on plastic combination will be necessary.
Even with this combination of materials, prosthetic geometries involving fully or partially constrained hinges, or ball in socket configurations in which impingement of the two components occur within the range of movement which is likely to be used by the patient, expecially where the ball is captive, are likely to generate shear forces at the cement bone junction which will lead to its breakdown, and subsequent loosening with progressive bone destruction.

iii) Spontaneous tightening under load if movement at the cement bone junction does start can only occur with a tapering intramedullary stem when the loads applied to it are compressive in the sense that the implant under load is tending to be driven into the medullary canal rather than twisted within the canal or withdrawn from it under tension. Minimal loosening under the latter two circumstances is likely to lead to progressive bone destruction

and gross loosening. Spontaneous tightening under load in effect is utilising a variant of the principle of the engineering taper; for it to be effective, the stem, and the configuration of the medullary canal must possess tapering sections. The latter should have a somewhat elliptical outline so that resistance may be offered to torsional stresses. The implications of the phenomenon of tightening under load are considerable: spontaneous tightening under load must be at times, or perhaps always, involve cracking of the acrylic cement mantle around the stem. Provided however that such cement is well constrained physically, it is still capable of highly effective load transmission, and will continue to be so as long as repetitive movement of cement against bone does not destroy the bone and thus the effective surrounding constraint. The ability to tighten prevents repetitive movement.

The role of the surgeon

6.   It is perhaps superfluous to state that the surgeon employing acrylic cement should be familiar with the mechanical properties of the material, and the way these are influenced by the total environmental circumstances surrounding the implant. What is more important is that the surgeon should appreciate the ways in which he can make the most of the mechanical properties of the acrylic cement he is to use, and to realise that he has under his control the capacity to at least double or halve the effective mechanical properties of the acrylic he is using. Detailed consideration of these matters is out of place here: suffice it to say that, in order to make the most of the mechanical properties of acrylic cement, the surgeon should:
 mix the cement dough with a slow beating frequency
 minimise the formation of laminations, voids and porosities by early placement of the cement, with, if possible, pressurisation of the cement both before and after placement.
 minimise the inclusion of blood and tissue debris by adequate cleansing of the bone surface, and by the achievement of haemostasis, together with the use, where appropriate of a cement syringe.
 employ the cement in situations where it is physically fully constrained by bone of 'good' quality.
 avoid the use of prosthetic components with stress raising features such as sharp corners and edges.

Achievement of implant fixation - the upper limb

7.   To what extent can the foregoing be applied to the upper limb?
The use of intramedullary stems in the upper limb immediately runs into difficulties related first to the size of the medullary canals. With the exception possibly of the upper end of the humerus, reaming the medullary canals in the upper limb for the reception of intramedullary stems is virtually certain to involve reaming down to cortical bone throughout the whole or part of the medullary canal. This produces a smooth surface on which acrylic cement can get no grip and furthermore devascularises $\frac{2}{3}$ of the cortex. The dimensions of the canals also make for difficulties in filling with cement, though with the judicious use of syringes, these can be overcome. The loads applied to intramedullary stems in the elbow, and to a lesser extent in the fingers, comprise a substantial torsional and even tensile elements, especially where the stem is associated with a fully or partially constrained hinge. This combination of circumstances is likely to lead to excessive shear stresses at the cement bone interface, leading to failure with movement at the interface. Such movement is likely to be repetitive for spontaneous tightening under load is impossible

with this loading pattern; thus, progressive bone destruction and gross loosening is the sequel, as seen in Fig. 3. Imperfect filling of the canal, voids and laminations in the cement, together with stress raising features on prosthetic components may lead to cement cracking which will compound the problem.

8. Fixation of prosthetic components to the scapula presents special problems owing to a relative lack of bone stock, especially where the use of geometries involving captive heads may lead to high cement-bone interface stresses at the extremes of movement. Once again, bone preparation may involve the exposure of a cortical surface, and spontaneous tightening under load is impossible, so that once movement starts, it is likely to be progressive, with bone destruction.

9. Thus, one is brought to consideration of surface replacement with totally unconstrained components. Even with such replacements in the upper limb, the sizes and shapes of the surfaces to be replaced, the limited areas of cement-bone contact, and the uncertain loading patterns, do not allow unguarded optimism with regard to the prospects of long term stability using acrylic cement.

Conclusions

10. The use of bone cement for implant fixation in the various joints of the upper limb can be summarised as follows:

i) The shoulder joint. Intermedullary fixation in the humerous should be satisfactory, but there are grave doubts as to the suitability of the glenoid or scapula. The loads may well be tensile, there is only a small area for achieving fixation and there may be no trabecular bone left for the cement to extrude into.

ii) The elbow joint. Preparation of the medullary canal in the ulna will leave a smooth cortical tube, that is devascularised. The cement will prevent endosteal revascularisation. The cavity is hard to fill with cement and it is very difficult to insert the stem of a prosthesis centrally in the medullary canal. Tension and torsion loads cannot be resisted.

iii) The finger joints. The same drawbacks as for the elbow joints.

iv) The wrist joint. At the present time other operations are far superior to total replacement of the wrist joint.

Two final points need emphasis.

It is a mistake to look upon acrylic cement as a sort of universal 'bone glue' which will work as well at all joints as it does when properly used at the hip. The principles of its use suggest that in many situations in the upper limb, it is inherently unsuitable for the local conditions, and premature failure of fixative can be anticipated.

Many patients requiring prosthetic replacement in the upper limb are suffering from polyarthritis such that they require the assistance of their upper limbs to manipulate crutches, etc. for walking. This type of activity may impose entirely unnatural loads upon upper limb replacement prostheses, and has to be considered when decisions concerning surgical replacement in the upper limb are being made.

REFERENCES

1. McKee G.K., Watson Farrar J. Replacement of arthritic hips by the McKee Farrar prosthesis. JBJS 1966, 48B, 245

2. Harris W.H., Schiller A.L., Schollar J.M., Freiberg R.A., Scott R. Extensive localised bone resorption in the femur following total hip replacement. JBJS, 1976, 58A, 612

3. Miller J. Paper given at the sixth combined meeting of the Orthopaedic Associations of the English Speaking World. London, September 1976.

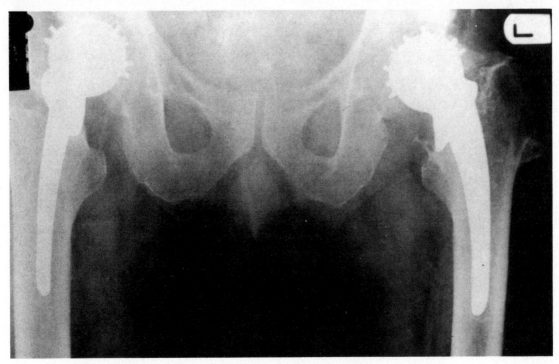

Fig. 1: Bilateral hip arthroplasty of a 72 year old man, performed in 1965

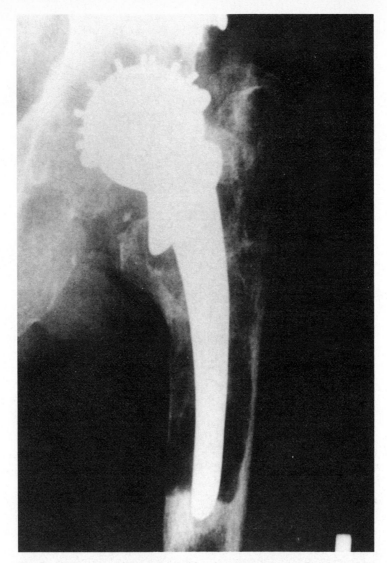

Fig. 2: Marked bone destruction in hip of patient shown in Fig. 1, after 7 years

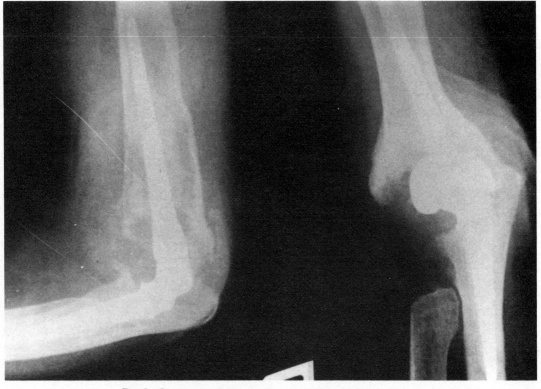

Fig. 3: Gross bone destruction in a total elbow joint

C156/77

A BIOMECHANICAL ANALYSIS OF ELBOW JOINT FUNCTION

A.C. NICOL, BSc, N. BERME, BSc, MSc, PhD, J.P. PAUL, BSc, PhD, ARCST, CEng, FIMechE
Bioengineering Unit, University of Strathclyde

SYNOPSIS. A three dimensional biomechanical analysis of elbow joint function is presented. Eating, dressing, pulling a heavy object and assisted standing from the seated position were investigated. The external force measurements were made using a six component load transducer in conjunction with displacement measurements using multiple cine-cameras. Cadaveric studies were made relating to the position and orientation of the major load bearing structures. The equilibrium equations were solved to assess the joint loadings taking into account the relevant constraint conditions. During the dressing and eating activities compressive loads of 300N were calculated to be acting on both sides of the trochlear notch. The joint load reached peaks up to 1700N in the other activities.

INTRODUCTION

1. The relatively high success rate of total joint replacements in the lower limb, in the recent years, has encouraged both surgeons and manufacturers to undertake design and development of joints for the upper limb. Of the major load bearing joints of the upper extremity, the elbow has received most attention since disability at this joint effectively prevents most of the functions of normal daily living. Earlier designs of replacement endoprostheses for the elbow utilized a hinge to replace the humero-ulnar articulation. The fixation of the prostheses to both bones was achieved by stems cemented into the medullary cavities. A follow-up of such joint replacements, however indicated that the failure rate at the interface between bone and stem was unacceptably high and this phenomenon occurred at the humeral interface (Ref.1.) The more recent elbow prostheses include a variety of new designs. A preliminary assessment of these also indicates that the problems associated with the arthroplasty of the elbow are by no means satisfactorily solved.

2. Previous investigations of elbow joint function have involved estimations of the performance of arm muscles during controlled movements. Hunsicker (Ref.2) performed a series of strength tests for various arm positions and directions of applied effort but did not analyse the loadings on any of the anatomical structures. Work by Groh (Ref.3) and Simpson (Ref.4.) involved the estimation of the forces acting across the elbow joint during simple tasks such as pure elbow flexion. The load sharing between humero-radial and humero-ulna articulations has been studied by Halls and Travill (Ref.5) Pressure transducers were inserted into the joint spaces of fully extended cadaveric arms and the long bones were loaded axially. They reported a load sharing of 57% and 43% between the radius and the ulna respectively. The excision of the interosseous membrane did not alter the results. Walker undertook further experimental studies to investigate the behaviour of the various load bearing structures under similar test conditions (Ref.6)

3. A rigorous biomechanical analysis of the elbow to establish design criteria for joint replacement was long overdue. This paper presents the resultant load actions transmitted between the forearm and the upper arm in various activities, and assesses the loadings on the articular surfaces, ligaments and the tendons.

METHOD

4. When a patient undergoes joint replacement surgery the aim of the operation is to restore function as close to 'normal' as possible in addition to minimizing the pain. However, establishing the range of movement and loading to be characterized as 'normal' is not so straightforward as in the lower limb, where the activities to be restored are standing and locomotion.

5. When pain is relieved it should be expected that the patient will utilize his arms to their maximum capability which will be limited by the condition of his other joints and his muscular power - although it must be recognized that muscular regeneration may well occur. Therefore, it can be expected that the patient will not only undertake moderate activities like eating or dressing but also use his arms in such activities as assisting rising from a chair or sitting up in bed, pulling a table or even lifting a heavy object. These activities may be performed in varying patterns by each patient and this adds to the complex nature of the total range of activities to be analysed.

6. In this study three young, healthy male adults were used as test subjects. Naturally, the data obtained from the 'healthy' groups of subjects would yield information in the conservative range for establishing design criteria. It is also desirable to study the loading patterns for the patients suffering from joint disorder and also the ones who have had joint replacement. Test results obtained from all three groups would be relevant to the study of the endoprostheses design. However an understanding of the normal function of the joint was considered essential before the disabled groups were studied.

7. To determine the load actions transmitted between the forearm and the upper arm both the position of the extremity in space and the loads acting distal to the joint need to be known. The former was achieved by filming the

subject simultaneously from three directions. The directions selected were front, back and the side of the investigated arm. The cine-cameras were driven by synchronous motors at a speed of 50 frames/s. The anatomical landmarks of the arm were identified by markers attached to the body as shown in Figure 1. From these markers the direction cosines relative to a ground reference system of the co-ordinate axes relating to the humerus and ulna were calculated.

8. The forces that act on the forearm are the reactions between the hand and the environment, and the gravity and inertia forces corresponding to the accelerations of the hand and forearm. The loads acting on the hand were monitored by incorporating a transducer into the environmental system, e.g. the arm rest of the chair used for the assisted seat rise. The strain gauged transducer was capable of measuring all six quantities describing the externally applied loads. The measurements taken were sampled synchronously with the cine-cameras.

9. The accelerations of the arm were calculated from the displacement data by using a suitable universal double differentiation technique (Ref.7). This information together with the standardised mass properties of the hand and the forearm and where relevant the object held, yielded the inertia loading acting on the elbow. During the activities which involved only inertia loadings a mass of 1 kg was carried in the hand to simulate the actual situation.

10. The activities that were studied had to be standardized to a certain degree to avoid totally random movements and to make a comparison between the subjects possible. For both the eating and dressing activities the movements adopted were those used by physiotherapists to mobilise patients for these activities. During the assisted seat rise the subjects were asked to keep their legs extended to ensure active weight bearing by the arms as shown in Figure 2. The table pulling exercise was performed from a seated position with the arm supinated. A table having a mass of 40 kg was pulled on a vinyl floor by flexing the elbow from a fully extended position.

11. During all these activities the EMG signals from the biceps and triceps were monitored to determine the periods during which these muscle groups were active.

12. Cadaveric measurements were taken to assess the lines of action of the forces developed in the main load bearing structures of the elbow. By comparing the internal structural measurements with the external dimensions of the dissected arms scaling factors were calculated. These factors were used to determine the position of the relevant load bearing structures of the test subjects from external measurement relating to anatomical landmarks.

ANALYSIS

13. The humero-ulnar articulation is primarily a hinge joint whose idealized shape can be described as two semi-frusta of cones joined at their smaller diameter. The smooth curved contour of the articulation allows very small rotations of the humerus relative to the ulna orthogonal to the main flexion axis. This mechanism permits the collateral ligaments to bear load without loss of effective contact at the articulation. Figure 3 shows the radius and the ulna and the diagrammatic representation of the ligaments, the tendons of the muscles triceps, biceps and the co-ordinate axes system attached to the ulna. The

line between the centres of the coronoid and olecranon processes was taken as the y-axis. The positive direction for the flexion axis (z-axis) was taken laterally for the right arm, and medially for the left one. The direction of the x-axis was obtained for a right handed co-ordinate system. The flexors brachioradialis and brachialis though not shown in the figure were included in the analysis. The three flexors were assumed to share load proportional to their effective cross sections as described by Bankov and Jorgensen (Ref.8).

14. For a series of instants in time at intervals of 20 ms during each activity equilibrium equations were solved taking into account the relevant constraint conditions and the load values. First the moment about the flexion axis was taken to be balanced by either flexor or extensor loading depending on its direction These muscles are not confined to a plane normal to the flexion axis. Therefore, any muscle activity had an effect on the values of the moments in the directions orthogonal to the flexion axis as well as the forces in all three directions. These had to be modified prior to further calculations. This approach of calculating the forces transmitted by the load bearing structures as determined from their major functional requirements was adopted throughout this analysis. For this reason a step by step solution method was more appropriate to use as opposed to solving all relevant equations simultaneously.

15. The moment about the y-axis together with the force in the x-direction determined the compression in the x-direction on the trochlea. If this compressive force on the medial and/or lateral side of the articulation was calculated to be negative this indicated loss of joint contact at that section. To achieve equilibrium the necessary tensile force must then be transmitted by the appropriate ligament(s). Similarly, a simultaneous solution of the moment in the x and y-directions respectively gives the values of the force components in the y-z plane. The force acting on the radial head was also included in these equations. The solution to these latter set of equations modified the forces transmitted by the ligaments. Therefore the complete solution could only be obtained after a series of iterations.

RESULTS AND DISCUSSION

16. Figure 4 shows the forces transmitted by the elbow joint and the variation in elbow angle during the dressing acitivity. As the arm was simultaneously abducted and flexed to an outstretched position the elbow angle varied from 95° to 150° where it remained for half a second before returning to the starting value. During this activity the net moment about the elbow-flexion axis was balanced by tension in the flexor muscles. The magnitude of biceps force varied as shown between 0 and 135 N. The medial ligament was loaded during most part of the activity with an occasional minimal loading of the lateral ligament. Both sides of the trochlear notch were loaded throughout the activity where resultant compressive forces of 300N were encountered. Compression on the radial head was not very significant. It was present for a brief period and reached 150N.

17. The duration of the dressing activities for the three subjects ranged from 1.6s to 2.1s However, the magnitude of the accelerations and therefore the forces transmitted in each case were consistent.

18. Results of the forces transmitted by the elbow joint

during the eating activity were found to be of the same order of magnitude as those reported for the dressing activity. In both groups of tests the fluctuation in muscle activity corresponded to the gross movement of the arm. It was noted that muscle stimulation was reduced during lowering of the arm due to gravitational effects. However, at the end of the descent phase substantial braking efforts were produced by the opposing muscle group.

19. For the assisted seat rise, the elbow angle increased from 95° to 170° as the subject raised himself to the fullest stretch of the arms (see figure 4). The figure also shows the forces transmitted by the elbow joint. During the initial stages of the elbow movement the elbow flexors were active, however, triceps activity became dominant after the elbow angle exceeded 120°. The tension in the triceps muscle reached 240N as the arm approached the fully extended position. Throughout the activity the tension in the lateral ligament was of the order of 500N whereas the medial ligament transmitted no load. Since the humero-radial joint was also redundant the resultant medial joint force was greater than that experienced on the lateral side. Figure 5 shows that peaks of 1700N and 800N occurred on the respective joint surfaces during the maximum tension in the triceps.

20. During the table-pull exercise the elbow angle was decreased from 145° to 85° as shown in figure 6. The motive power was provided by the flexor muscles where the tension in the biceps gradually decreased from 650N to zero. Tension of 1900N in the medial ligament was characteristic of this strong flexor activity since the biceps insertion is lateral to the joint centre. The resulting compressive forces on the two joint surfaces and the humero-radial joint follow patterns which are similar to the muscle forces.

21. Two of the subjects (body masses 65 and 75 kg) completed the seat rise activity in approximately one second, whereas the third subject (body mass 65 kg) took twice the time. However, from Figure 7, it can be seen that the duration of major muscle activity was of the same order of magnitude. The forces developed in the joint for all three subjects were also comparable.

22. The duration of the table-pull activity showed little variation between subjects. Figure 8 shows the pattern of biceps force versus time. Following initial peaks of similar magnitudes the muscle force gradually decreased to zero. Two of the force patterns showed a close relation with each other whereas the magnitude of the muscle force developed by the third subject was significantly higher. The magnitude of the loads transmitted to the hand of this subject indicated higher rotational moments in the direction of pull, which accounts for the increased muscle force. The joint forces for this subject were also correspondingly higher.

23. All the activities analysed were standardized to ensure repeatability and to enable comparisons to be made between subjects. The constant mass carried in the hand during the eating and dressing activities provided a close control on the inertial force actions. However, for activities involving hand contact with the environment no control could be exercized over the degree of isometric effort utilized. This resulted in variations between subjects in the joint loads for a standard activity.

24. The myoelectric signals from biceps and triceps muscles indicated some degree of antagonistic muscle

activity during tests involving hand contact with the environment. This effect was mainly due to the involvement of the shoulder complex, and was not included in the present analysis. Consequently, the calculated values represent the minimum loadings transmitted by the elbow joint.

REFERENCES

1. Souter, W.A. Arthroplasty of the elbow; Orthop., Clin. of N. America; 1973, Vol 4, No. 2, 395-413.

2. Hunsicker, P.A. Arm strength at selected degrees of elbow flexion. WADC Tech. Report. 54-548, 1955, Aug. Project No. 7214.

3. Groh, H. Proceedings I. Elbow fractures in the adult. Biomechanics of the elbow joint. Hefte Unfallheilkd, 1973, 114; 13 - 20.

4. Simpson, D. An examination of the design of an endoprosthesis for the elbow. M. Sc. Thesis, University of Strathclyde, Glasgow, 1975.

5. Halls, A A. and Travill, A. Transmission of pressures across the elbow joint. Anat. Rec; 1964, Vol 150, 243-248.

6. Walker, P. S. Personal communication, 1975.

7. Andrews, B. J., Ph.D. Thesis (in preparation). University of Strathclyde, Glasgow 1976.

8. Bankov, S., and Jorgensen, K. Maximum strength of elbow flexors with pronated and supinated forearm. Communications from the Danish National Association for Infantile Paralysis, 1969, No. 29.

APPENDIX : JOINT EQUILIBRIUM

The analysis of the equilibrium of joint surface and elbow joint structures was undertaken when all the external forces and moments acting on the forearm were calculated in terms of the axes previously defined (See Figure 3). Equilibrium was established by the action of muscle, ligament and joint forces on the ulna and radius.

The resulting system of unknown parameters was made statically determinate by grouping certain muscles together; by analysing the various patterns of ligament function; by simplifying the articular surfaces of the elbow joint to those having geometrically specified contours; and by considering the constraint conditions that muscle and ligament forces cannot be compressive whereas the joint force cannot be tensile.

Five unknown quantities were defined: one muscle group force, one ligament force, and three joint forces or one muscle group force, two ligament forces and two joint forces. The computations were executed in three stages:

1. Muscle Forces

Assuming negligible joint friction and zero antagonistic muscle action, tension in the flexor or extensor muscles was obtained from the equation of moments about the z − axis. To model the actual effect of the flexor muscles, the assumptions of Bankov and Jorgensen (Ref.8) were adopted i.e. the tensions in biceps brachii and brachialis were assumed equal while the tension in brachioradialis was taken as half the tension in biceps brachii. Either flexor or extensor function was selected depending on the sign of the net moment about the z − axis of the elbow joint.

2. Ligament Tensions

The medial and lateral ligament tensions (T_M and T_L) were derived from the simultaneous solution of x − direction equilibrium equation ($\Sigma F_x = 0$) and the y − axis moment equilibrium equation ($\Sigma M_y = 0$). The medial and lateral joint forces (R_M and R_L) in the x − z plane were also calculated:

Double Ligament Action : The initial condition considered both ligaments to be loaded simultaneously. In such cases the joint forces in the x − z plane were both zero and this produced a 'joint gap'.

Single Ligament Action : In the majority of cases the tension in one ligament or the other was calculated to be negative, indicating that the particular ligament was not carrying load. Single ligament action was subsequently considered and the choice of medial or lateral ligament tension was determined by the direction of the resultant moment about the y − axis. Positive values produced a toppling effect on the humerus in the x − z plane which created tension in the medial ligament (T_M) and a compressive joint force (R_L) on the lateral articular surface of the trochlear notch. The equations $\Sigma F_x = 0$ and $\Sigma M_y = 0$ enabled the solution for T_M and R_L.

Single Ligament − Double Joint Force : When the ligament force was small compared to the joint force, equilibrium was obtained by simultaneous load bearing of medial and lateral joint surfaces. The equilibrium equations were modified accordingly to cater for this condition.

3. Joint Forces

The remaining joint forces in the y − z plane were calculated using equilibrium equations obtained from the summation of force actions in the y −direction and the summation of moments about the x − axis. It was found that two resultant joint forces were sufficient to provide equilibrium for all force actions in the y − z plane and were defined 'positive' when acting on the superior surfaces of the trochlear notch (+ y direction). Contact between the trochlea and the inferior surfaces of the trochlear notch produced negative values for force on the medial side of the joint and a compressive force on the head of radius on the lateral side of the assembly. The two simultaneous equations $\Sigma M_x = 0$ and $\Sigma F_y = 0$ containing the unknown quantities were solved to complete the initial analysis for joint equilibrium.

In certain cases the solution to these equations modified the forces transmitted by the ligaments and therefore called for an iterative procedure for a complete solution.

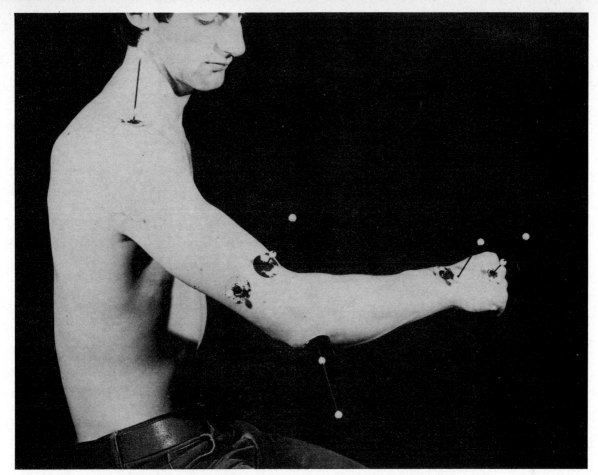

Fig. 1: Marker system used during photography

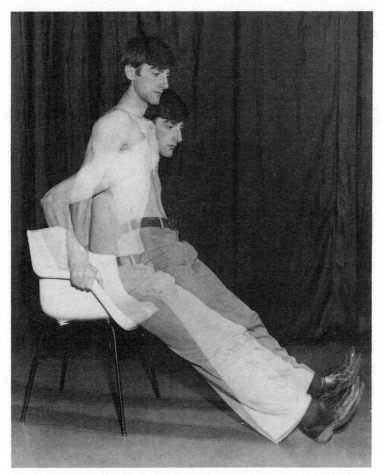

Fig. 2: Movement involved in the 'seat-rise' activity

49

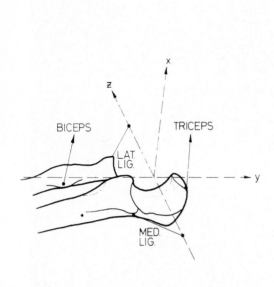

Fig. 3: Definition of joint axes and load carrying structures

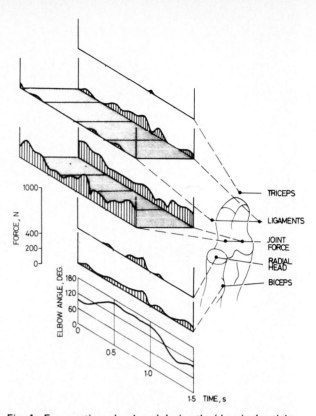

Fig. 4: Force actions developed during the 'dressing' activity

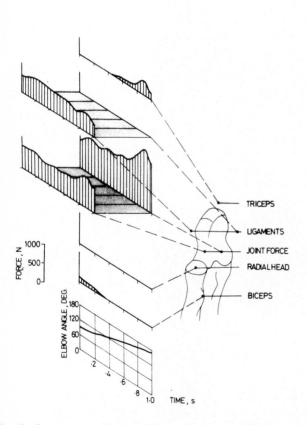

Fig. 5: Force actions developed during the 'seat-rise' (Subject 3)

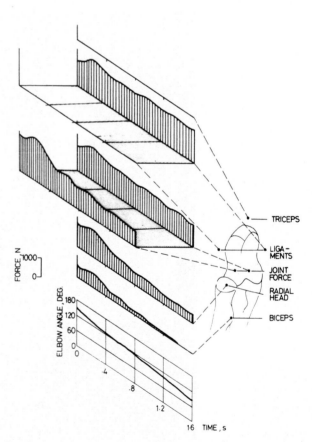

Fig. 6: Force actions developed during the 'table pull' (Subject 1)

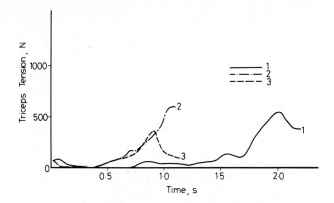
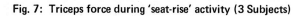
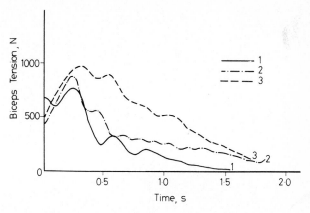

Fig. 7: Triceps force during 'seat-rise' activity (3 Subjects)   **Fig. 8: Biceps force during 'table pull' activity (3 subjects)**

THE EVOLUTION OF THE STANMORE HINGED TOTAL ELBOW REPLACEMENT 1967-1976

J.T. SCALES, FRCS, CIMechE
Institute of Orthopaedics (Univ. of Lond.), RNO Hospital, Stanmore

A.W.F. LETTIN, MS, FRCS, BSc
RNO Hospital and St. Bartholomew's Hospital, London

I. BAYLEY, FRCS
Institute of Orthopaedics (Univ. of Lond.), RNO Hospital, London

Satisfactory excision arthroplasty of the elbow is impossible and arthrodesis unsatisfactory, if more than the articular surfaces and the immediately adjacent bone is removed. When more extensive resection of the distal humerus or proximal ulna is necessary to eradicate disease in these bones, the resulting defect must be bridged by bone grafts or better still, a prosthesis which might usefully incorporate an artificial joint to provide stable, pain free movement.

In 1967 work began at the Institute of Orthopaedics to design a prosthesis which would not only bridge such a defect but could also be used in the treatment of arthritis and complicated fractures affecting the elbow joint.

Mechanism of the Elbow

The elbow joint has humero-ulnar and humero-radial articulations and the joint cavity is continuous with the superior radio-ulnar joint. The three articulations together forming the cubital articulation.

Movement at the elbow joint, that is the articulation between the humerus and the ulna and the humerus and the radius, is essentially flexion about a fixed axis passing through the centre of the trochlea. The axis of rotation is oblique to both the long axes of the humerus and the forearm and so results in a carrying angle which may vary between $10-15^\circ$ in the male and $20-25^\circ$ in the female with the elbow in full extension. The range of flexion varies between $140-160^\circ$ from the fully extended to the fully flexed position in the normal joint. Sometimes a few degrees of hyperextension may be possible and a few degrees of axial rotation of the ulna may occur at the extreme of flexion and extension range, but true pronation and supination occurs only at the radio-ulnar joints.

The stability of the elbow joint is largely due to the shape of the humero-ulnar articulation, which permits hinge movement without lateral displacement. Lateral stability of the joint is aided by the radius. The concavity of the head articulating with the capitulum of the humerus, although configuration of the joint suggests the primary function of the humero-radial articulation is to stabilise rotation of the radius on the ulna.

A secondary function is the transmission of load to the humerus under high or instantaneous loading sparing the humero-ulnar joint and perhaps preventing damage. It is difficult to determine the magnitude of load transmitted through the head of the radius to the capitulum because axial forces acting on the distal end of the radius are transmitted to the ulna through the interosseous membrane.

It is probable that under normal conditions minimal load is transmitted through the humero-radial joint and the fact that the head of the radius can be removed without causing major residual disability supports this hypothesis.

The elbow joint as a whole however, must be considered a weight bearing joint. Not only resisting abnormal forces encountered in falling, for example, but also transmitting part of the body weight in patients with a stick or crutches.

Design Study

When the initial studies to design a replacement for the elbow and the adjacent bone began in 1967, it was considered advisable to attempt to replace the entire cubital articulation for the following reasons. Such a design was thought more likely to restore the anatomy and function of the elbow and provide greater stability than the humero-ulnar prosthesis alone.

The prosthesis was required to transmit loads which might develop when a patient used crutches and to withstand sudden shock loads which might be encountered in a fall.

It should be possible to restore a normal range of flexion and extension, supination and pronation.

The prosthesis must be stable throughout its range of movement.

The carrying angle between the long axes of the upper arm and forearm must be reproduced.

Fixation to the adjoining bone must be secure.

The materials used in construction of the prosthesis must not induce undesirable local, distal or general, tissue reactions.

The surgical technique and the instruments required to introduce the prosthesis must not be complex.

The dimensions of the prosthesis must be such that the soft tissues are free from pressure throughout the range of movement.

A salvage procedure must be possible in those cases where only the joint is replaced.

The initial prosthesis, Fig.1, consisted of a

humeral component which replaced the trochlea and the capitulum with an intramedullary stem set at 8° to the axis of rotation. The ulnar component was recessed into the humeral component and also had an intramedullary stem set at 8° to the axis of rotation. Thus when the components were assembled there resulted a carrying angle of 16° between the long axes of the components. This of course, necessitated separate right and left prostheses.

The intramedullary stem of the ulnar component was preset to a shape that would fit the intramedullary cavity without adjustment providing it was reamed to 8 mm diameter. The long axis was so placed that it lay 8 mm posterior to the long axis of the humeral components when the components were assembled.

The radial component was also set at 8° to its intramedullary stem and was surmounted by an ultra high molecular weight polyethylene RCH 1000 (1) articular disc with a central hole. This disc articulated with the capitulum. The extended axle of the humero-ulnar articulation which ran in RCH 1000 flanged bushes, carried a pivot pin which projected through a slot in the capitulum and into the hole in the RCH 1000 'head' of the radial component. In this manner the radial component was allowed to flex and at the same time rotate.

To introduce the prosthesis the humerus was transected through the condyles approximately 25 mm from the articular surface at an angle of 8° to its long axis in the frontal plane.

The olecranon notch was excised in order to introduce the ulnar component. The major part of the olecranon process together with the triceps insertion was retained. The coronoid process was trimmed as far as the radial notch. The head of the radius and the adjacent bone were removed but the tuberosity was not disturbed.

This prosthesis was 45 mm wide, 24 mm long without the stems, and 22 mm from front to back. The axis of the intramedullary stem of the humeral component was 8 mm anterior to the axis of the ulnar intramedullary stem.

The prosthesis was implanted into the cadaver using a pneumatic gun to introduce the acrylic cement into the medullary cavities of the bones. It proved extremely difficult to align and assemble the individual components correctly. Movements, especially pronation and supination resulted in undue stresses on the fixation of the components in the bone.

Mark 1 Prosthesis

As a result it was concluded that a simpler prosthesis was required abandoning the radial component. This enabled the dimensions of the 'body' of the prosthesis to be reduced with consequent preservation of bone, and in particular the humeral condyles could be preserved and the prosthesis recessed between them. The redesigned joint, Fig.2, was made of airmelt/aircast cobalt chromium molybdenum alloy (2). Because the humeral component was completely recessed between the condyles, the axle could no longer be passed through the prosthesis to assemble the two components after they had been individually cemented into place. The overall length of the prosthesis made it impossible to introduce it in one piece. The hinge assembly was therefore made an integral part of the humeral component and the stem of the ulnar component was secured to the remaining part of the prosthesis after insertion, by expanding a hollow rivet - A in Fig.2.

The first joint of the basic design was used in February 1969 in a 29 year old man (3) with a flail left elbow resulting from the explosion of a land mine. The neurovascular supply to the forearm and the hand was intact, but a previous arthrodesis had failed because of sepsis, followed by extrusion of the bone grafts.

After warning the patient of the possible complications which might follow elbow replacement the prosthesis was adapted to provide a lower humeral and proximal ulna replacement.

After the operation progress was at first satisfactory and within five weeks the patient could extend the elbow fully and flex to 95° with 20° of pronation and almost full supination.

Nine weeks after the operation however, a sinus developed from which Staphylococcus was isolated. Eventually after extensive antibiotic therapy and plastic surgery the prosthesis was removed. There was considerable fibrosis which helped stabilise the elbow and with a moulded leather splint reasonable function was restored.

Mark 2 Prosthesis

Soon after the design of the Mark 1 prosthesis had been completed, it was decided to modify the bearing of the elbow joint to incorporate ultra high molecular weight polyethylene RCH 1000 bushes in the ulnar component. The existing cobalt chromium alloy castings could not be modified, so the humeral and ulnar components were machined from Titanium 160 (4). Because of the unsuitable wear characteristics of Titanium 160, cobalt chromium molybdenum alloy bushes were press fitted into the humeral component. The hinge was assembled prior to operation, by expanding the ends of the hollow axle, Fig.3, and the main proximal and distal components were assembled as before.

The first elbow of this type was inserted in October 1970 with considerable improvement in function and lasting pain relief, Fig.4. This patient's condition is summarised (Elbow 1) in tables 1 and 2 which report the results of the standard non-modified total elbow replacements.

A modified Mark 2 prosthesis was made at the same time (1970) for a patient (5) with a giant cell tumour, involving the whole of the medial part of the lower end of the left humerus and invading the adjacent soft tissue. In this case it was possible to assemble the components at the hinge at operation.

In August 1976 this patient had no pain and 85-135° of flexion with full pronation and supination. The skin over the olecranon was normal in appearance, and was not tense on full flexion.

This modified prosthesis is not included in the

overall analysis of results (tables 1 and 2) and other individually made variations of the standard design are similarly excluded but are mentioned in the text where appropriate.

Mark 3 Prosthesis

The relative displacement of the axes of the humeral and ulnar intramedullary stems was increased to 15 mm in the Mark 3 prosthesis, Fig.5, to increase the range of movement of the elbow without causing undue compression of the soft tissues anterior to the joint.

The assembly of the components at operation was also simplified by incorporating the hinge in the distal or ulnar component. This part of the prosthesis was then joined to the intramedullary stem of the humeral component after both had been separately inserted, with a bolt passing from the posterior to the anterior aspect of the prosthesis.

A prosthesis of this design but with a modified ulnar component was made for a 27 year old woman (6) who had sustained a compound fracture of the right elbow at the age of eleven. Over the years various operative procedures had been carried out including excision of the proximal end of the ulna, which was followed by a wound infection. In February 1970 a McKee elbow prosthesis had been inserted. The humeral component became loose in June 1970. In September 1970 the humeral component was recemented, but by March 1971 it had become loose once more. Several blood examinations revealed a moderate eosinophilia and the patient was allergic to Penicillin, iodine and adhesive plasters. There was no clinical evidence at this time of infection, but in June 1971 the McKee prosthesis had to be removed. No organisms were grown from wound swabs or from the prosthesis.

The modified Mark 3 prosthesis was inserted and three weeks after the operation the elbow had regained a range of flexion from 45-100° with 30° of supination and 45° of pronation.

Unfortunately, the patient developed pain once more, and in December 1974, three and a half years after the operation, patch testing revealed sensitivity to cobalt and nickel, elements present in the hinge part of the prosthesis. The humeral component was loose but the ulnar component remained firmly fixed.

In January 1975 a fluctuant swelling developed over the point of the elbow. This was aspirated on several occasions and Staphylococcus albus organisms were cultured from the aspirate, so the prosthesis was removed.

It was difficult to determine whether the failure of the procedure was due to a primary low grade infection present before the insertion of the Stanmore prosthesis, a metastatic infection, sensitivity to cobalt and nickel or a combination of infection and sensitivity to elements in the cobalt chromium molybdenum alloy.

In January 1973 another modified prosthesis was used in a patient (7) who had sustained a compound comminuted fracture of the elbow, with gross loss of bone, two years earlier. The wound had been infected following injury, but at the time the prosthesis was implanted there was no clinical evidence of infection. Post operatively however, the wound never completely healed and the prosthesis had to be removed because of infection in July 1975.

Mark 4A Prosthesis

Because of the problems associated with the manufacture of the humeral component in commercially pure Titanium Type 160, the Mark 3, Fig.5, was redesigned in cast cobalt chromium molybdenum alloy, Fig.6. A bolt-type lock for the humeral stem was used and the bearing was all cobalt chromium molybdenum alloy. The intramedullary stems of both components were made of Titanium alloy Type 318 (8) (6%Al., 4%V.). By the time the prosthesis had been redesigned it had been decided to use only metal plastic bearings so no prosthesis of this type was used in a patient.

Mark 4B Prosthesis

The Mark 4A was modified by boring out the ulnar component and fitting polyester Hostadur KVP 4022 (9) bushes. The resulting Mark 4B prosthesis, Fig.6, was used in three patients between August and October 1971 (table 1 and 2). Subsequent work however, in the Institute of Orthopaedics, showed that Hostadur KVP 4022 would degrade in the body and so its use was discontinued. Although some wear of the bushes has occurred, which can be detected clinically, so far this has been of no consequence to the patients.

It is interesting to note that one patient (No.2 table 2) fell and fractured the neck of her humerus on the same side as the prosthesis four months prior to assessment. The fracture healed and there was no evidence of prosthetic loosening.

Mark 5 Prosthesis

The method of assembling the two components of the Mark 4B prosthesis was still not satisfactory in clinical practice. Repeated trial reductions with the prosthesis in place may be necessary to determine the correct position of the components before they are finally cemented into place. Each time the prosthesis must be assembled and then taken apart.

The Mark 5 prosthesis, Fig.7, was designed to take advantage of the resilience of RCH 1000 polyethylene. Slotted bushes were fitted into the humeral component which enabled the ulnar component carrying the axle to be snapped into position when the elbow was flexed to 90°. The components were assembled at the axle once more and the prosthesis was still recessed in the bone of the lower end of the humerus. The RCH 1000 bushes acted as bearings for the ulnar component and the flange faces of these bushes as thrust washers between the ulnar and humeral components. All the metal components were of Titanium alloy Type 318 (8) and were anodised.

A simple screw operated disarticulation instrument hooked over the humeral component and enabled the ulnar component to be pushed out of the slotted RCH 1000 bushes when the elbow was flexed to 90°. The ulnar components could be readily withdrawn from the marrow cavities of the respective bones.

Six elbows of this type were used and the results are included in tables 1 and 2, although two patients (Nos. 7 and 8) now live abroad and personal follow up has been impossible. It is understood however, that both patients have functioning elbows. Because of the inadequate data they have not been included in the overall summary of results.

One joint (No.9) (tables 1 and 2) became loose for no obvious reason and was removed two years after insertion and so the assessment (table 2) is the assessment of the salvage procedure. The elbow was still much better than it had been before the prosthetic replacement.

Mark 6 Prosthesis

Since January 1975 the Mark 6 prosthesis, Fig.8, has been in use. The design is essentially the same as the Mark 5 but the humeral stem is shorter and no longer has the acrylic cement retention depressions , shown in Fig.7. The metal components are made of vacuum melt/vacuum cast cobalt chromium molybdenum alloy (10) rather than Titanium 318 and four elbows of this type are included in this review. One was removed (No.12) after five months because of loosening, thought to be the result of Staphylococcus infection. Even so the patient was no worse after the salvage procedure than he had been pre-operatively.

Operative Technique

The operative technique has evolved as a result of work on the cadaver and operative experience in clinical practice. Briefly, the elbow joint is exposed through a posterior approach after turning down a tongue of triceps muscle based on its olecranon attachment. The remaining part of the triceps on either side is reflected anteriorly, if possible in continuity with the common flexor and extensor origins. The ulnar nerve is transposed anteriorly and the head of the radius is resected. The collateral ligaments are divided and the posterior capsule excised to allow the joint to be dislocated. The tip of the olecranon is removed flush with the base of the trochlear notch, preserving the triceps attachment.

The medullary cavity of the ulnar is located with a small Patons burr and gradually enlarged with flexible reamers of increasing diameter until it is large enough to accept the stem of the ulnar component (6 mm). If the size of the ulna permits, 7 or 8 mm reamers should be used for part or the full length of the ulnar stem. The mouth of the medullary cavity should be enlarged a further 1 to 2 mms. A shallow groove in the floor of the trochlear notch is developed proximally from the opening of the medullary canal.

A small triangle of bone is removed with nibblers from the centre of the trochlea with its apex at the apex of the olecranon fossa where the medullary cavity of the humerus can be located with the Patons burr. The medullary cavity can usually be prepared to take the prosthesis with curettes and the use of reamers is rarely required.

The triangle between the condyles is gradually enlarged with bone nibblers, until it is large enough to accept the humeral component of the prosthesis, the bearing of which should lie at the level of the epicondyles.

Several trial insertions of the components, at first separately and later assembled may be required before the correct position for the final insertion is achieved. The prosthesis is in the correct position when there is no relative movement of the components in the humerus and ulna, when the elbow is moved through the flexion-extension range. The coronoid process of the ulna may need trimming and the anterior capsule may need to be excised to allow full extension. Osteophytes and any residual articular cartilage should be nibbled away from the humerus and the ulna especially if there is a tendency to impinge one on the other.

Acrylic cement can only be satisfactorily introduced into the medullary cavities of the humerus, and especially the ulna with a syringe or gun with a 12 cm long nozzle. The cement must be of a creamy consistency (e.g. Simplex C) (11) in order to pass through the nozzle. Great care must be taken to prevent the semi-liquid cement from escaping from the medullary cavities into the wound. The two components are inserted at the same time when the cement is in a 'pastry-like' state, and are immediately assembled. The elbow is held extended until the cement is set. The wound is closed with suction drainage and immobilised post operatively until the wound has healed.

Salvage Procedure

With all total joint replacements an acceptable salvage procedure must be possible, and in two patients in this series (Nos. 9 and 12) the prostheses have been removed. Because the humeral condyles and the major part of the olecranon are retained, the latter can be trimmed to fit between the condyles after the prosthesis and the cement have been removed. This results in a stable pseudarthrosis with a good functional pain free range of movement.

The Present Design

The Mark 6 prosthesis appears to meet the criteria which were formulated nine years ago. It is constructed of cobalt chromium molybdenum alloy (10) with RCH 1000 (1) bearings, materials which rarely induce undesirable tissue reactions. It is easily introduced and removed with the minimum of special instruments and a satisfactory salvage procedure is possible. There are right and left sided prostheses allowing a carrying angle between the upper arm and the forearm. The ulnar component is 10.5 cm long and the humeral component is 13 cm long, and the intra-medullary stems allow secure fixation within the marrow cavities. The overall width of the joint is 20 mm allowing the humeral component to be recessed between the humeral condyles. The ulnar component is 7 mm wide and this can be recessed within the retained portion of the olecranon. The relative antero-posterior displacement of the axes of the humeral and ulnar intramedullary stems has remained at 15 mm. There is no pressure on the soft tissues throughout the range of movement.

The axis of rotation of the prosthesis can be made to coincide with the axis of rotation of the elbow joint, making a normal range of stable movement possible. The prosthesis appears to withstand the loads it would normally be expected to bear and in suitable patients restores a functional range of pain free movement.

(1) RCH 1000 - Registered Trade Mark of Ultra
High Molecular Weight Polyethylene, manufactured
by Ruhrchemie, Oberhausen-Holten, W. Germany.

(2) Chemical composition of the alloy complying
with that specified in BS 3531 Part 1 1968.

(3) Patient of Mr. J.N. Wilson, Royal National
Orthopaedic Hospital, Stanmore, England.

(4) Commercially pure Titanium manufactured by
Imperial Metal Industries (Kynoch) Limited,
Birmingham, England.

(5) Patient of Mr. R.S. Sneath, The Royal
Orthopaedic Hospital, Birmingham, England.

(6) Patient of Mr. D.M. Brooks, Royal National
Orthopaedic Hospital, London, England.

(7) Patient of Mr. L. Trickey, Royal National
Orthopaedic Hospital, Stanmore, England.

(8) Titanium alloy Type 318, manufactured by
Imperial Metal Industries (Kynoch) Limited,
Birmingham, England.

(9) Hostadur KVP 4022 - a polyethylene
terephthalate polymer, manufactured by Farbwerke
Hoechst AG, 6230 Frankfurt (Main) 80.

(10) Alivium - Trade Mark for vacuum melt/vacuum
cast cobalt chromium molybdenum alloy. Supplied
by Zimmer G.B. London, U.K. and complying with
the relevant specifications in ASTM 75, 1967
and BS 3531 Part 1 1968.

(11) Surgical Simplex is the trade name of acrylic
bone cement,manufactured by Howmedica
International Ltd., (N. Hill Plastics Division),
49 Graylins Road, London, N16 OBP, England.

ACKNOWLEDGEMENTS

We wish to acknowledge the staff of the Department
of Biomedical Engineering, in particular Mr. P.H.
Ansell, Mr. P. Child and Mr. J.D. Wood, who have
been concerned intimately with various aspects
of the development of the work. We also wish
to acknowledge the assistance given by Mr. S.
Medcraft, Metallo Medical Limited, Swindon, who
has also contributed a great deal of thought and
effort. We wish to acknowledge the grant from
the Department of Health & Social Security which
has made possible various aspects of the work.

| | | | | | | | TABLE 1 | | | |

ELBOW NO.	NAME	R/L	MARK NO.	DISEASE	DATE INSERTED	CONDITION AT TIME OF REVIEW SEPTEMBER 1976
1	A.T.	R	2	R.A.	10/70	SATISFACTORY
2	H.C.	L	4B	R.A.	8/71	SATISFACTORY
3	G.Mc.	R	4B	R.A.	9/71	SATISFACTORY
4	G.O.	L	4B	R.A.	10/71	SATISFACTORY
5	G.Mc.	L	5	R.A.	11/72	SATISFACTORY
6	G.O.	R	5	R.A.	11/72	SATISFACTORY
7	J. de S. (Portugal)	R	5	OLD T.B.	11/72	PT. LOST TO F/U PROSTHESIS REMAINS IN SITU.
8	A.W. (Brazil)	R	5	POST TRAUMA	5/73	PT. LOST TO F/U PROSTHESIS REMAINS IN SITU.
9	A.E.	L	5	R.A.	1/74	REMOVED 3/76 ULNA COMP. LOOSE, STERILE ON CULTURE
10	B.C.	R	5	R.A.	7/74	SATISFACTORY
11	U.S.	R	6	R.A.	1/75	SATISFACTORY
12	F.S.	R	6	R.A.	3/75	REMOVED 8/75 ULNA & HUM. COMP. LOOSE ? INFECTION.
13	B.C.	L	6	R.A.	5/75	SATISFACTORY
14	H.Y.	R	6	R.A.	5/75	SATISFACTORY

TABLE 2

PAT. NO.	PAIN		RANGE OF MOVEMENT						PATIENT ASSESSMENT
	PRE.OP	POST OP	FLEXION-EXTENSION			PRONATION-SUPINATION			
			PRE.OP	POST OP	% CHANGE	PRE.OP	POST OP	% CHANGE	
1	S	N	$40^{\circ}-140^{\circ}$	$50^{\circ}-120^{\circ}$	−30	$80^{\circ}-140^{\circ}$	$15^{\circ}-165^{\circ}$	+150	I.G.
2	S	M	$60^{\circ}-120^{\circ}$	$35^{\circ}-160^{\circ}$	+108	$0^{\circ}-180^{\circ}$	$10^{\circ}-180^{\circ}$	−6	I.G.
3	MO	MO	$60^{\circ}-100^{\circ}$	$40^{\circ}-150^{\circ}$	+175	$70^{\circ}-95^{\circ}$	$60^{\circ}-90^{\circ}$	+20	I.G.
4	S	M	$45^{\circ}-130^{\circ}$	$60^{\circ}-145^{\circ}$	0	$45^{\circ}-135^{\circ}$	$10^{\circ}-160^{\circ}$	+67	I.
5	MO	N	$90^{\circ}-125^{\circ}$	$40^{\circ}-170^{\circ}$	+271	$60^{\circ}-100^{\circ}$	$60^{\circ}-120^{\circ}$	+50	I.G.
6	S	M	$45^{\circ}-170^{\circ}$	$40^{\circ}-135^{\circ}$	−24	$15^{\circ}-135^{\circ}$	$0^{\circ}-180^{\circ}$	+50	I.
7	M		NOT REVIEWED						
8	MO		NOT REVIEWED						
9	S	N	$80^{\circ}-100^{\circ}$	$40^{\circ}-100^{\circ}$	+200	$70^{\circ}-130^{\circ}$	$90^{\circ}-140^{\circ}$	−17	I.G.
10	S	N	$75^{\circ}-100^{\circ}$	$20^{\circ}-160^{\circ}$	+460	$90^{\circ}-100^{\circ}$	$70^{\circ}-170^{\circ}$	+900	I.G.
11	S	N	$65^{\circ}-125^{\circ}$	$35^{\circ}-160^{\circ}$	+108	$60^{\circ}-115^{\circ}$	$50^{\circ}-180^{\circ}$	+136	I.G.
12	S	MO	$45^{\circ}-135^{\circ}$	$25^{\circ}-140^{\circ}$	+27	$45^{\circ}-180^{\circ}$	$0^{\circ}-180^{\circ}$	+33	S.
13	S	N	$60^{\circ}-120^{\circ}$	$30^{\circ}-160^{\circ}$	+116	$60^{\circ}-90^{\circ}$	$50^{\circ}-140^{\circ}$	+200	I.G.
14	S	N	$40^{\circ}-140^{\circ}$	$40^{\circ}-160^{\circ}$	+20	$20^{\circ}-180^{\circ}$	$0^{\circ}-180^{\circ}$	+13	I.G.

KEY S = Severe
MO = Moderate
M = Mild
N = None

Average Gain Degrees 42°
Average Gain Per cent 119%

Average Gain Degrees 42°
Average Gain Per cent 133%

KEY
I.G. Improved Greatly
I. Improved
S. Same
W. Worse

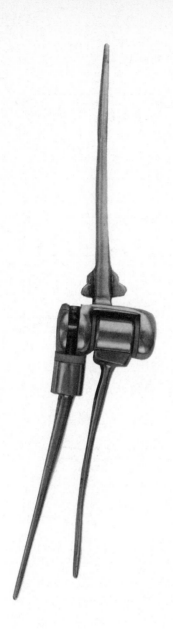
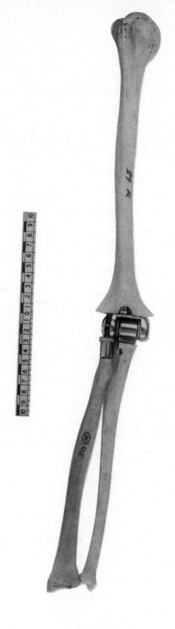

Fig.1:

Mк. 1.   Mк. 2.

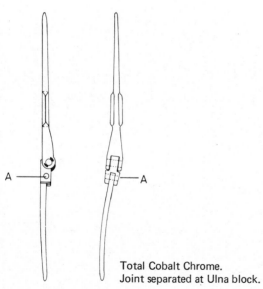
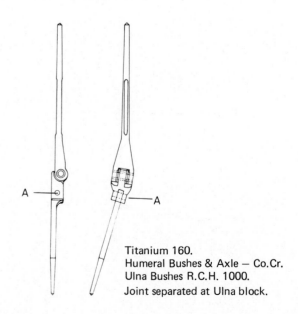

Total Cobalt Chrome.
Joint separated at Ulna block.

Titanium 160.
Humeral Bushes & Axle — Co.Cr.
Ulna Bushes R.C.H. 1000.
Joint separated at Ulna block.

Fig. 2:   **Fig. 3:**

60

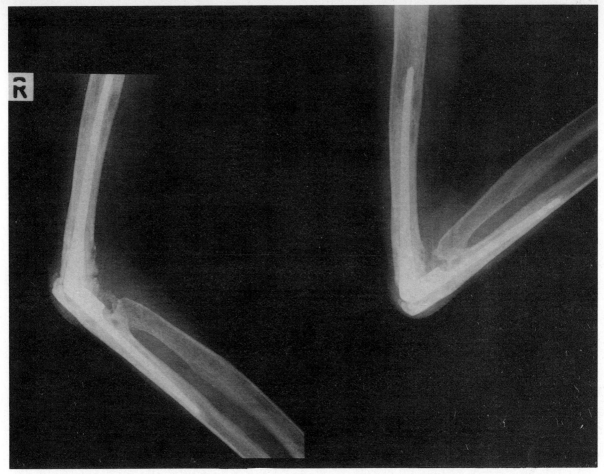

Fig. 4: Patient 1. Components of prosthesis secure in humerus and ulna. Flexion — extension range 70°. Has no pain

Mκ. 3.

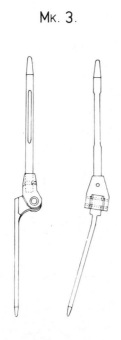

Titanium 160.
Humeral Bushes & Axle — Co.Cr.
Ulna Bushes R.C.H. 1000.
Joint separated at Humeral block.

Fig. 5:

Mκ. 4 A & B.

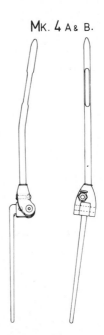

4A.   Humeral Pin — Ti.318
      Humeral Block, Bolt & Axle — Co.Cr.
      Nut — Co.Cr. Nylock.
4B.   As 4A. but with Ulna Bushes of Hostadur 4022.
Joint separated at Humeral block.

Fig. 6:

MK. 5

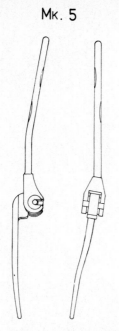

Titanium 318.
Axle — Co.Cr.
Bushes — R.C.H. 1000.

Fig. 7 :

MK. 6.

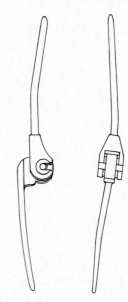

Co.Cr.Mo. alloy   vacuum melt-vacuum cast.
R.C.H. 1000   Polyethylene-Bushes

Fig. 8:

FLEXIBLE ELBOW JOINT REPLACEMENT

R. W. PRITCHARD, MD

INTRODUCTION

1.   Long term success with the total hip joint and more recently the total knee joint arthroplasties have led to the development of prosthetic implants for the major joints of both the upper and lower extremeties. Advanced degenerative disease of the elbow joint is a painful and disabling condition which, until the advent of joint replacement surgery, remained un-treated for the most part. Synovectomy and radial head excision often improve elbow function, but do little to deal with the instability and pain relating to advanced destructive changes at the ulna-humeral articulation. The unpredictable and often disappointing results following fascial arthroplasty of the elbow (Ref. 1,2) have encour-aged investigators to develop a prosthetic im-plant for this joint. Early attempts to replace the elbow joint centered around the use of the rigid metallic hinge prosthesis. These protheses were generally bulky in size and required the resection of a significant amount of bone from the distal end of the humerus or proximal ulna. Using these early restrained hinges, excellent post-operative results could be predicted as long as long as meticulous surgical technique was employed (Ref. 3). Long term follow-up studies of the restrained hinge type elbow pros-thesis have indicated an alarming degree of loosening of the intra-medullary fixation (Ref. 4, 5, 6). Pain, bone fracture and instability are not infrequently encountered as the sequela of stem loosening.

2.   The propensity of the restrained elbow prosthesis to loosen its intramedullary fixation in spite of the use of methyl methacrylate cement is most likely related to its inability to accommodate to torque forces transmitted onto its component parts as axial rotation of the forearm occurs. Early anatomical studies by Fick (Ref. 7) and a more recent three dimension-al study by Morrey and Chao (Ref. 8) have rep-orted axial rotation of the forearm and abduct-ion-adduction motion patterns at the ulna-humeral articulation during flexion of the elbow. Since the restrained hinge prosthesis cannot abduct, adduct, or rotate as does the normal elbow joint, forces which would otherwise be absorbed at the joint level by the supporting soft tissues are instead transmitted across the axis of the hinge onto the medullary stem fix-ation, the weak link of the system. Long term stressing of the bone cement junction leads to erosion of the bone matrix lining the medullary canal and ultimate loosening of the stem fix-ation occurs.

REQUIREMENTS FOR THE OPTIMALLY DESIGNED ELBOW PROSTHESIS

3.   In theory, the short comings ascribed to the restrained hinge prosthesis should be over-come by employing a semi-restrained prosthetic design. Such a prosthesis would provide adequate stability to combat the distraction forces working at the joint level. Abduction, adduction and rotational capabilities of this design would reduce stress on the intra-medullary fixation of the components parts through the dissipation of torque forces onto adjacent soft tissue structures at the joint level (i.e. collateral ligaments, joint capsule, surrounding muscles and tendons). Several points should be considered when design-ing a prosthesis for optimal function in addition to the importance of the semi-restrained features. The size of the prosthesis must be considered. Bulky components will necessitate the sacrifice of more bone than desirable from the distal humerus or proximal ulna. If arthrodesis should be required as a salvage procedure in the face of an infected prosthetic implant., such an operation will be twice as difficult if the bone stalk has been sacrificed at the time of the original implant surgery. In addition, if the epicondyles of the humerus are sacrificed as is required with the Dee prosthesis the stabilizing effect of the med-ial and lateral collateral ligaments is lost. The components should be small enough so that they will fit within the bony confines of the distal humerus and proximal ulna. Since a minimal amount of soft tissue exists on the posterior aspect of the elbow joint, ulceration of the skin by exposed metallic edges of the prosthesis may result when its component parts are not completely encased by the bone. This occurs more frequently when resec-tion of the proximal portion of the olecranon process is required for insertion of the prosthesis. In this situation the posterior soft tissue is particularly vulnerable to ulcerating pressure when the joint is held in a position of flexion as occurs for example when the forearm is rested upon a table top. If ulceration of the skin develops, the joint becomes immediately suscept-ible to deep infection. Length of the intra-medullary stem should be an important design consideration. Theoretically, a long stem would transmit forces of stress over a greater surface area than a shorter stem and thus be less likely to loosen in its fixation. The prosthetic parts should be fabricated from bio-compatible materials with a low wear potential, such as high molecular weight polyethylene and stainless steel.

MATERIAL

4.   Adhering to the concepts of the optimal
design, a semi-restrained polyethylene and stainless steel hinge was developed (Fig.1). (A non-
hinged design was rejected because of the need for
greater inherent stability of the prosthesis when
used in patients with severe flexion contractures
or marked bone and soft tissue destruction). The
polyethylene component was designed with a 20 degree anterior angulation of its distal portion in
order to conform with normal joint anatomy. The
ulna component, composed of stainless steel, has
an 8 degree valgus angulation built into its intramedullary stem, thus necessitating a right and
left version. Reduced stem sizes for both ulna and
humeral components were fabricated in order to
accommodate small medullary canal sizes. When
articulated, the ulna and humeral components bear
weight on their respective articulating surfaces.
The semi-restrained effect is accomplished by a
loose fit between these two component parts, thus
giving the joint a 5 degree axial rotation as well
as an 8 degree abduction-adduction capability. A
polyethylene axle with a reinforced stainless steel
center core is employed to prevent distraction of
the two components. The axle was designed with a
self locking snap fit and is inserted at the time
when the humeral component is cemented into place.
The prosthesis can be inserted after a minimal
amount of bone has been resected. This is important if an arthrodesis is required at a later date.
The prosthetic components are completely encased
within the bony contours of the distal humerus and
proximal ulna (Fig. 2) thus negating the possibility of soft tissue irritation or ulceration by
sharp edges of the components.

TECHNIQUE OF OPERATION

5.   With the patient in a supine position and a
sand bag under the scapula, the involved elbow is
positioned across the chest. A posterior incision
is made from the distal one-third of the humerus
and curved across the olecranon process to the
proximal one-fourth of the ulna. A careful dis-
ection of the ulna nerve is carried out distally
until the motor branch to the flexor carpi ulnaris
is identified. Articular branches to the joint
are sacrificed and the ulna nerve is retracted out
of the surgical field using a one-half inch Penrose
drain. The tendon of the triceps muscle is incised
at the muscular tendonous junction using a V-shaped
incision. The apex of the V should lie at the
level of the olecranon fossa. If lengthening of
the triceps tendon is required due to a long standing extension contracture, this can easily be
accomplished at the time of soft tissue closure by
using a "V-Y plasty" technique. The tail of the
triceps tendon, now freed, is temporarily sutured
down to the dorsal portion of the proximal ulna
for better visualization of the joint. The
olecranon fossa is debrided of fat and synovial
tissue and the collateral ligaments are incised
just distal to their point of origin from the
medial and lateral epicondyles. These ligamentous
structures should be preserved since they will be
re-sutured at the close of the procedure adding
increased stability to the prosthetic joint. The
joint capsule is now freed along its medial and
lateral insertions onto the olecranon process and
the joint is flexed so that the articular surfaces
are fully visualized. A sharp osteotome is used
for excision of the radial head taking care to
preserve the annular ligament. If the annular

ligament is excised or if too much of the neck
of the radius is removed, the proximal radius
will subluxate when the elbow is actively flexed.
This subluxation which is caused by the unre-
strained pull of the biceps tendon gives the
patient a somewhat unpleasant and occasionally
painful snapping sensation as he flexes his
elbow. Once the radial head has been removed, a
reciprocating saw is used for excising the
articular surfaces of the olecranon by making
right angle cuts. Cancellous bone below the
articular surface of the olecranon is curetted
out and an opening is established into the medullary canal of the proximal ulna. Once opened, the
canal is reamed with a hand reamer or long stemmed
burr fitted into an air-driven power drill. The
mouth of the canal must be reamed sufficiently
wide in order to accept the prosthesis stem. It
may be necessary to transversely resect one-half
centimeter off of the tip of the coronoid process
in order to facilitate insertion of the ulna portion of the prosthesis. Reaming of the medullary
canal of the ulna must be carried out in a gentle
fashion since the cortical bone is thin, particularly in the rheumatoid patient, and easily
broached with the reamer. (Should the cortex be
penetrated by the reamer, a small piece of finely
woven stainless steel mesh may be placed within
the medullary canal against the defect in order
to prevent extrusion of methyl methacrylate into
the soft tissues of the forearm when the ulna
component is inserted.). A trial fitting of the
ulna component is carried out. If the medullary
canal of the proximal ulna is particularly small,
as in female patients, a small stem ulna component
should be chosen. Using the reciprocating power
saw, a transverse cut is made across the distal
end of the humerus preserving the epicondyles but
resecting a portion of the capitellum and trochlea.
A two centimeter width bone wedge is then resected
out of the remaining trochlea. The apex of the
wedge is extended through the olecranon fossa
into the medullary canal of the distal humerus.
The medullary canal is enlarged with a small bone
rongeur until a humeral reamer one-half inch in
diameter can be inserted into the canal. Once the
humeral canal has been reamed, a trial fit of the
polyethylene component is carried out. This
component may be trimmed to size with a power burr
if the medullary canal is small. A trial fit with
both components in place is carried out in order
to ensure that full extension and flexion of the
joint may be obtained. If full passive extension
is not possible more bone must be resected from
the distal end of the humerus. A capsulotomy of
the anterior joint capsule may also be required
in this situation. A small batch of methacrylate
cement is mixed and inserted into the medullary
canal of the ulna prior to impacting the ulna
component into place. A number of small notches
are cut into the polyethylene component with a
sharp scalpel to improve its fixation in the
methacrylate cement plug. Once again the methacrylate is mixed and inserted into the medullary
canal of the humerus with a cement syringe. The
polyethylene component is inserted approximately
80% of its length into the medullary canal and
articulated with the ulna component. Care should
be taken to insert the humeral component in the
correct orientation in terms of its anterior and
posterior surfaces. If the humeral component is
inserted with an incorrect anterior-posterior
orientation, the joint axis will be located 20
degrees posterior to the long axis of the humerus
and post-operative flexion will be compromised.

Once the two component parts have been articulated, the snap-fit axle pin is inserted and impacted into place with a special clamp. At this point, the humeral component is forced the remaining 20% of its length into the medullary canal so that the polyethylene condyles lie well supported on either side by epicondylar bone. Any methacrylate cement which has extruded into the anterior aspect of the joint should be removed so as not to act as an obstacle to flexion post-operatively. The collateral ligaments and joint capsule are carefully re-approximated using strong durable suture material. The triceps mechanism is re-anastomosed with similar material, carrying out a tendon length-ening if required. Hemovac drains are placed in the deep and superficial aspect of the wound after the ulna nerve is replaced in its anatomic position in the ulna groove. The subcutaneous fascia and skin are closed with re-absorbing suture material and a bulky dressing applied with a posterior plaster splint keeping the elbow in full extension. Post-operatively, intravenous antibiotics are used routinely for a period of 48 hours following which oral antibiotics are continued until wound closure is complete. The Hemovac drain is removed 48 hours after surgery. The bulky dressing and splint are removed four to five days after surgery and active motion of the elbow instituted. Discharge from the hospital is usually accomplished five to seven days after surgery with the arm restrained in a sling. Active exercises for the hand, elbow and shoulder are carried out by the patient at home or in the Outpatient Therapy Department on a daily basis. The use of an external support such as a crutch, cane, or walker is not discouraged if required due to other joint involvement in the lower extremities. The patient is advised against lifting objects weighing more than ten pounds and the fragile nature of the implanted prosthesis is impressed upon the patient prior to his leaving the hospital.

RESULTS

6.   Twentyfive patients with severe degenerative osteoarthritis of the elbow joint underwent implant-ation of the described semi-restrained hinge prosthesis. The patient age ranged from 28 years to 78 years with an average age of 62 years. The presenting complaint in 16 of the 25 patients was pain, unrelieved by mild analgesics. Two of the remaining 9 patients presented with the chief complaint of instability and the remaining 7 presented with an ankylosed joint. Seventeen patients (11 female - 6 male) suffered from diagnosed rheumatoid arthritis with multiple joint involvement. Eight patients (6 male - 2 female) developed degenerative elbow disease secondary to trauma. The average pre-operative range of motion of the involved elbows measured 35 degrees. In grading the post-operative results, a standard elbow analysis form was employed (Fig. 3). Range of motion, presence or absence of pain, stability and forearm strength were evaluated. The period of post-operative follow-up ranged from 24 to 36 months. Eighteen of the elbows were graded as excellent (score of 85 or greater) and showed an average pain free range of motion of 110 degrees with hand to face capability. Five elbows were graded as good (score 65 to 85) and two elbows were graded as poor (score less than 65). Compar-ison of the scoring for the good and excellent group showed the major difference to be in the range of motion capability of the elbow post-operatively. A review of the operative notes showed that full extension was not achieved at the operating table with these five patients. The two poor results followed fracture of the distal end of the polyethylene humeral component when it was used without supporting epicondylar bone. In one case, the medial epicondyle was present but a non-union of the lateral epicondyle existed. One year after the initial surgery both patients under-went removal of the fractured humeral component and re-insertion of a reinforced metallic humeral component. Now one year following their second surgery, both patients have full pain free range of motion and are rescored as excellent results. Roentgenographs of the twentyfive cases followed to date have shown no evidence of stem loosening in either the ulna or humeral components.

CONTRAINDICATIONS

7.   Use of the polyethylene humeral component when it is unsupported by bone due to the absence of the epicondyles is contraindicated. Fracture of the condylar portion of the prosthesis from the main part of the stem has occurred when used with-out adequate bone support (Fig. 4). A reinforced metallic humeral component has been designed for this situation (Fig. 5). This component retains the same lateral and rotary motion capabilities as does the all polyethylene humeral component. It has been used successfully by the author over the past sixteen months in patients with failed fascial arthroplasties or previous implant surgery. The operation should not be contemplated in the face of dormant or active infection of any parts of the elbow joint. If excessive scarring of the soft tissue about the elbow is present as a result of previous injuries, caution should be employed since a much greater likelihood of post-operative wound difficulties exists. Strong consideration should be given to the physical requirements that may be placed on this prosthetic joint by the patient. Use of the prosthesis in a manual laborer desiring to return to work, or in a physically active young person is contraindicated. Arthrodesis is the operation of choice in such situations.

CONCLUSION

8.   Long-term loosening of intra-medullary stem fixation following the use of restrained hinge prostheses in the elbow joint has prompted the developments of a semi-restrained hinge implant. This prosthesis was designed in accordance with the theoretical requirements for an optimal elbow design. It is the feeling of the author that the semi-restrained design of this prosthesis allows for dissipation of torque forces onto the support-ing soft tissue at the joint level which is responsible for the lack of stem loosening to date.

REFERENCES

1.   D'Aubigne, R.M. and Kerboul, M.: Les
Operations Mobilisatrices Des Raideurs Et Ankloses
Coe. Rev. Chir Orthop. 52:427, 1966

2.   Knight, R.A. and Van Zandt, I.L.; Arthroplasty of the Elbow. J. Bone and Joint Surg.,
34A:610, 1952.

3.   Dee, R.; Total Replacement Arthroplasty of
the Elbow for Rheumatoid Arthritis. J. Bone
and Joint Surg., 54B:88-95, 1972.

4.   Souter, W.; Arthroplasty of the Elbow.
Orth. Clinics of N. Amer., Vol. 4, No. 2, April
1973.

5.   Sledge, C.; Experiences with Total Elbow
Arthroplasty; Recent Developments in Total Joint
Replacement, Miami, Fla., December 1975.

6.   Bryan, R.; Technique and Experiences with
Total Elbow Prostheses. Recent Developments In
Total Joint Replacement. Miami, Fla., December
1975.

7.   Fick, R.; Handbuch der Anatomie und
Mechanik der Gelenke, unter Berücksichtigung
der Bewegenden Muskeln. Vol. 2, p. 299, Jena
1911.

8.   Morrey, B. and Chao, E.; Passive Motion of
the Elbow Joint. J. Bone and Joint Surg., 58-A,
No. 4, 501-508, 1976.

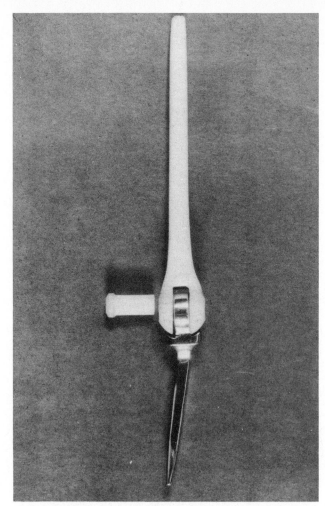

Fig. 1: Front view of the prosthesis with component parts
articulated

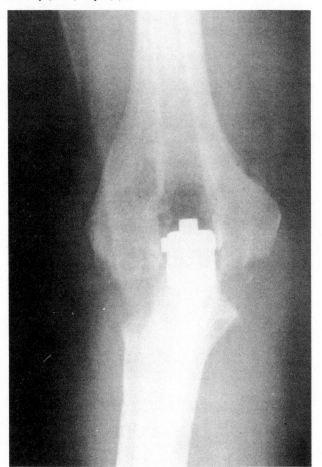

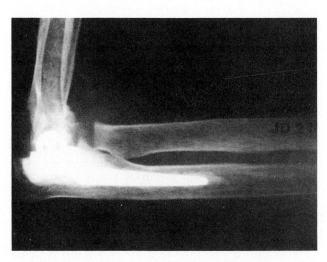

Fig. 2: Lateral post-oprative x-ray showing preservation of olecranon process, polyethylene humeral stem outlined by barium
impregnated methyl methacrylate cement. Also AP post-operative x-ray of implanted prosthesis showing the preservation
of medial and lateral epicondyles

PART I
RANGE OF MOTION

EXAMINATION	Pre-op	FU 6 mo	FU 1 yr	FU 2 yr	FU 3 yr
Date Examined					
The angle of greatest flexion					
The angle of maximal extension					
Difference: total elbow motion					

NUMERICAL RATINGS

	Pre-op	FU 6 mo	FU 1 yr	FU 2 yr	FU 3 yr
Difference: total elbow motion SCORE A					
Supination SCORE B					
Pronation SCORE C					

Score System:

Difference: total elbow motion	$<30^\circ$	$30-59^\circ$	$60-89^\circ$	$90-119^\circ$	$120-150^\circ$
Score	0	4	10	14	19

Extent of supination	$<30^\circ$	$30-60^\circ$	$>60^\circ$
Score	1	2	3

Extent of pronation	$<30^\circ$	$30-60^\circ$	$>60^\circ$
Score	1	2	3

PART II PAIN

EXAMINATION	Pre-OP	FU 6 mo	FU 1 yr	FU 2 yr	FU 3 yr
Date Examined		-			
DEGREE OF PAIN Score					
None 50					
Slight, with no compromise in activity 44					
Some mild pain after unusual activity 37					
Moderate, interfering with activity, requiring meds. 24					
Marked, with serious limitations of activity 10					
Complete disability 0					
SCORE D					

PART III STRENGTH

While the patient is seated, and his elbow rests on a table, he is asked to lift weights of 10, 5, and 2 pounds to a height of 6 inches above the table. At each examination, check the box which corresponds to the heaviest weight which the patient was able to lift to the prescribed height, and record the score on the double line at the bottom of the column.

EXAMINATION	Pre-OP	FU 6 mo	FU 1 yr	FU 2 yr	FU 3 yr
Date Examined					
PATIENT LIFTED Score					
10 lb 25					
5 lb 17					
2 lb 9					
0 lb 0					
Score E					

TOTAL FUNCTION SCORE
(Maximal score 100)

(Excellent 85-100, Good 65-84, Poor 64 or less)

Fig. 3: Post-operative elbow analysis form

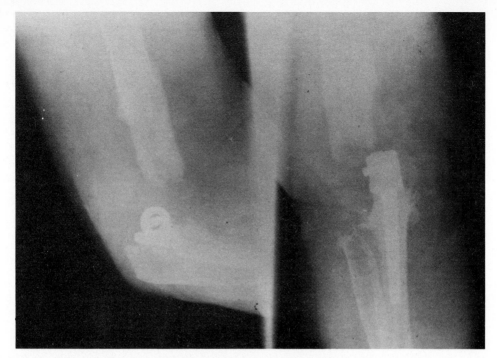

Fig. 4: AP and lateral x-rays of patient with fractured humeral component one year after implantation. (Note absence of supporting epicondylar bone)

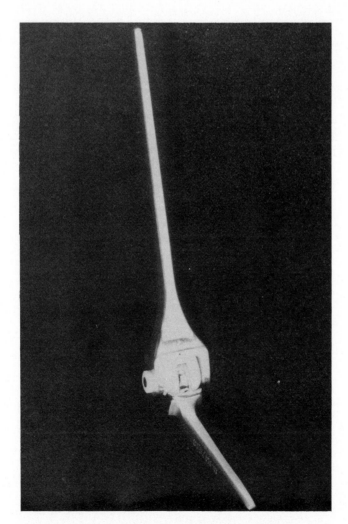

Fig. 5: Modified prosthesis with re-inforced long-stemmed metallic humeral component. Abduction, adduction, and rotational capabilities have been preserved

DISTAL HUMERAL PROSTHESIS FOR THE ELBOW

P. S. STEVENS, MD

SYNOPSIS   An elbow prosthesis has been designed, which replaces only distal humeral bone, and duplicates the shape of the intact distal humerus. It is of a single piece, does not use an intra-medullary nail, and requires no screws or other hardware to hold it in place. It is emplaced by a relatively simple surgical technique, and once emplaced is absolutely stable. It has been used in patients with varying types of elbow pathology over a ten year period, and the results in patients who do not have highly active rheumatoid arthritis or hemophilia have been excellent - it has been pain-free, stable, and provided an excellent range of motion.

The elbow as a joint for prosthetic emplacement

1.   In the past, the elbow joint has been considered one of the most satisfactory for arthroplasty. It might follow, therefore, that it is one of the most favorable joints for prosthetic replacement, and in fact, during the past few years numerous elbow prostheses have been designed.

2.   In humans, the important function of the upper extremity is to place the hand in the best position for use, and to move it from one location to another. A fused elbow causes severe disability by interfering with placement of the hand, while an unstable resected elbow limits the power of the hand and forearm.

Status of elbow prostheses ten years ago

3.   Prior to a decade ago all elbow prostheses were custom-made, and generally utilized intra-medullary nails, which tended to become unstable, and to alleviate this problem, the prostheses often had been provided with side plates, screws, and other hardware. Some were metal, some plastic and metal, some replaced only one side of the joint, while some were hinged, and replaced both sides. A search of the world literature revealed only a total of twenty-eight reported cases of prosthetic elbow replacement before 1967.

Conception of a new prosthesis, of unusual design

4.   In late 1966, Dr. Dana Street, an orthopaedic surgeon of international stature, presented a case of a patient who had an ankylosed elbow as a result of a car accident. At the time of the presentation, Dr. Street suggested that a prosthesis which replaced little humeral bone would be valuable - he felt it might be possible to make something of sheet metal which would 'snap on' over the distal humeral articular surface. Since that time, he and the author have been working in conjunction on the prosthesis which is the subject of this paper.

5.   At the outset, in attempting to design a new

prosthetic elbow, The author wished for the following: a) to avoid a total elbow, since it seemed that the elbow, being a non-weight-bearing joint, did not, in most cases, require a total prosthesis. b) to avoid a mechanical hinge joint, if at all possible; hinges, per se, with a pin in the center, are totally unphysiologic. The hinge, whatever it is made of, must wear. What happens to the wear particles? What lubri-cates the hinge? Does it not provide dead space for synovial reaction to occur, or for the accumulation of wear particles or bacteria? Is it not, by it's nature, quite rigid, not allowing a certain amount of flexibility in all directions, which all natural joints in the body do? c) to avoid an intramedullary nail. Intra-medullary nails, whether in the humerus, ulna, or both, will tend to become unstable with time, because of unusual forces acting on the elbow. Without attempting to describe these forces in detail here, it is sufficient to mention that intramedullary nails in elbow prostheses have, in fact, tended to become unstable to an unusual degree, so much so that some individuals advocate their abandonment in such prostheses. d) to make the prosthesis extremely simple, and of one piece only, not requiring any weldments, metal to metal or plastic to metal attachments, etc. e) to so design the prosthesis that it would, once emplaced, be absolutely stable on the bone, by its design alone, and not require the use of bone cement, screws, or other hardware. f) to design a prosthesis which replaced distal humeral bone only, and as little as possible, in case further procedures were required. g) to be inert. h) to provide a good range of motion, i) to eliminate dead space within the joint, j) to be manufacturable on a mass-production basis, and relatively simply so, so as not to be prohibitively expensive, and k) to design the prosthesis with the operative procedure in mind, so that the operation would be relatively simple and straight forward, so that no major muscle origins would be severed, so that the joint cap-sule need not be destroyed, and so that vital nerves and arteries were not exposed to undue hazard.

Universality of distal humeral shape

6. It was found, by the study of over a hundred x-rays of elbows, that the shape of the distal humerus is constant - in other words, there may be bigger or smaller distal humeri, but they all have the same basic shape. Thus, it was possible to come up with a formula for this shape, which would, if manufactured in prostheses of different sizes, fit all elbows well enough for adequate function. (Figure 1) This is a very simple formula, but it is the correct formula. Note that the diameter of the capitellum (C) is equal to the diameter of the trochlea (T), and that the distance from the lateral edge of the capitellum to the intracondylar hump (X) is also equal to the capitellar diameter. If one thinks about it, it makes perfect sense. If the diameters of the capitellum and trochlea were not identical the elbow would be a crooked joint-if the distance from the lateral edge of the capitellum to the intracondylar hump was not equal to the capitellar diameter, then the capitellum would not be a sphere, which it has to be for proper rotation of the radial head.

The prosthesis

7. Figure 2 shows the prosthesis.
Essentially the device is a cylinder, made of stainless steel or titanium, with a varying external contour that corresponds to the formula. The center of the cylinder is drilled out, and a keyway is milled along one side so that it opens into the central hole. The width of the keyway is less than the diameter of the central hole. Slightly inset on the capitellar end of the cylinder there is a sharpened, chisel-like edge surrounding the central hole. A driver fits into the central hole on the trochlear side, and has a shoulder which abuts against the medial end of the prosthesis. The articular surface of the prosthesis is polished to a mirror gloss and the inside surface is left rough as it was machined.

8. In principle the prosthesis works as follows: It is driven onto the trimmed distal end of the humerus in a lateral direction, the capitellar cutting edge acting as a shaping tool and providing a perfect fit. Once in place the prosthesis is immovable, and no screws or pins are required to maintain its position. It cannot move distally because the bone is thicker in the central hole than in the keyway, and it does not move laterally or medially because the roughly machined surface of the central hole provides numerous gripping places for the bone.

Sizes of prostheses, and means of selection

9. Of all the adults surveyed, none had an elbow prosthesis width of less than 1-1/2" or greater than 2-1/4". It was found that seven sizes of prosthesis, varying in width by 1/8" increments between these two limits, were sufficient to fit all elbows. For convenience in selecting the proper size of prosthesis it was found useful to make a transparent phototemplate, (Figure 3) supplied by the prosthetic manufacturer, on which were the outlines of the seven sizes of prostheses as viewed in their anteroposterior projection. The template is placed over an anteroposterior roentgenogram of the elbow to be reconstructed, or of the contralateral elbow of the same individual, if the architecture of the

elbow to be operated on is markedly altered. The size of prosthesis selected is the one which corresponds to the outline which gives the best fit. To select the best fit, the outline is placed midway between the subchondral surfaces of the humerus and radius-ulna complex, as seen on the roentgenogram. This line corresponds to the line of contact of the articular cartilage surfaces.

Operative procedure

10. The elbow is approached through a medial incision which is centered over the medial epicondyle and extended about two inches proximal and two inches distal to the epicondyle. The ulnar nerve is identified and retracted or otherwise protected from injury. A capsulectomy is performed, and in cases of ankylosis the ulna and radius are separated from the humerus. If articular cartilage remains on the ulnar joint surface, it is carefully spared. The end of the humerus is then delivered through the incision and a Kirschner wire is drilled into the trochlea along what is presumed to be the axis of the joint, being sure that the wire is not exactly perpendicular to the humeral shaft, but rather pointing a few degrees superiorly, as it is drilled in, since the carrying angle of the ulna on the humerus is about seven degrees abducted from the body.

11. The end of the humerus is then trimmed down with an osteotome, high speed burr, sabre saw, or oscillating power gouge (the last being the most rapid technique), keeping all cut surfaces parallel to the Kirschner wire. (Figure 4) When the end has been trimmed down sufficiently, the prosthesis is driven into place. Since the capitellar end of the prosthesis with its cutting edge performs the final shaping of the humerus as it is driven on, the distal end of the trimmed-down humerus is left slightly larger than the internal drilled out portion of the prosthesis. To avoid excessive trimming of the humerus, it was found useful first to trim only the most medial portion and then drive the prosthesis on a little way. When it is removed the mark left by the cutting edge serves as a guide for further trimming of the bone. This procedure is repeated several times as the trimming progresses.

12. For the final placement of the prosthesis, it is hammered on with the driver until the driver contacts the medial epicondyle (Figure 5); then the driver is removed, and the prosthesis is driven into final position using an impactor placed against the flat end of the prosthesis. Generally, the prosthesis is driven on until it lies approximately midway between the epicondyles (Figure 6), but an attempt is made to find the position which best restores the normal kinematics of the joint. As the prosthesis approaches its final position, it is helpful to articulate the ulna and radius with it periodically to find the ideal position. The groove in the prosthesis which articulates with the semilunar notch should be exactly even with the coronoid and olecranon fossae. If the prosthesis lies too far medial, the elbow may sublux later. If the prosthesis is driven too far laterally, it is extremely difficult to draw it back into position since it

grips the bone very tightly. If it is too far lateral, it is necessary to make an incision on the lateral side of the elbow, and drive the prosthesis back by hammering on its capitellar end, using the driver as an impactor. If the head of the radius is severely deformed, it is resected. The semilunar notch is also sculptured if necessary to make it articulate accurately with the prosthesis. It is often necessary to remove some of the coronoid process and the olecranon, to deepen the coronoid or olecranon fossae, or to do both procedures, if these structures interfere with normal flexion and extension. Once the proper relationships are established, the joint is reduced, and the wound closed in layers. The origins of the flexor muscle groups are re-attached on the epicondyles if they had been detached during the exposure. Transplanting the ulnar nerve forward is performed if indicated. A posterior molded splint, from palm to axilla, with the elbow in about forty-five degrees of flexion is applied until the soft tissues have healed, or for about ten days to two weeks, during which time isometric exercises are performed to tolerance. Active range-of-motion exercises are started after the splint is removed.

Results - stability

13. All of the prostheses of this design have been absolutely stable on the humerus - and our first patient was done ten years ago. (Figures 7 A, B, and C) There has been no tendency of the prosthesis to slip in any direction, in fact, dense new cortical bone grows inside the prosthesis, to better fix it in place. (Figure 8). Correspondence with others who have used the prosthesis have confirmed its total stability. In fact, we had an occasion, in one of our patients - case three in our original paper - (Journal of Bone and Joint Surgery, September 1974) - to remove the prosthesis; because of pain, which turned out not to be due to the prosthesis, and we found it almost incredibly difficult to remove - so firmly had the bone grown to the inside of the prosthesis. Also, it should be noted that after two years in the body, there was no evidence of synovitis, fluid, tissue reaction, or wear of the prosthesis. As a matter of fact we emplanted the prosthesis in a different patient, who is doing well at this time.

Strength of the bone in the keyway

14. Concerning the strength of the bone in the keyway: The patients in our case series have sustained falls on the elbows with the prosthesis and no fractures have occurred. From our correspondence with others who have used the prosthesis, there have been no fractures.

The body's tolerance of the prosthesis

15. The first two prostheses emplaced were made of type 316 stainless steel. There has been no evidence of reaction to the prosthesis. All others have been of titanium, because of it's greater inertness and lightness. Similarly, there has been no sign of reaction, inflammation, or rejection.

Wear of the prosthesis

16. Most of our cases were in individuals with total bony ankylosis, where there was no articular cartilage. Hence, we had to carve a new semilunar notch out of bone. In two cases, we have had to re-operate, one because of an error on our part in placement of the prosthesis, the other because of formation of fibrous scarring of the capsule. In each case, we found no significant wear of the prosthesis, and in fact, we found growth of fibrocartilage in the re-made semilunar notch, which served as the living articular cartilage.

Freedom from pain

17. We estimate that over a hundred of these prostheses have been emplaced in the past ten years worldwide. We have only emplaced eighteen ourselves. Nonetheless, we have been in communication with our colleagues, and I think we can report that this prosthesis is remarkably pain free. Of all the cases which have been done, of all the communications we have received, I can only report two cases which have had pain. One was recently done (two months ago), had osteomyelitis, now has mild pain with motion, and hopefully will improve. The other patient was, in this writer's opinion, mentally deranged. He had pain before the prosthesis, with the prosthesis, with a different prosthesis, with arthroplasty, with fusion, and he was finally admitted to a mental hospital for treatment of alcoholism and overuse of narcotics.

Ease of emplacement

18. After a little practice, and using an oscillating power gouge, the entire operation has been performed on an ankylosed elbow in an hour - no vital structures are damaged, only the medial capsule is incised, and only the medial flexor muscle origins must be cut and re-implanted on the medial epicondyle.

Elimination of dead space

19. No dead space exists, since the prosthesis only duplicates previously existing distal humeral surface.

Amount of bone resected

20. As mentioned previously, only a tiny amount of distal humeral bone has been removed, so if a different procedure should be desired later, (which, incidentally, has proved unnecessary) good humeral bone stock remains.

Simplicity

21. It is immediately obvious that this prosthesis is extremely simple, with no moving parts, etc. In particular, it has no hinge, and no intramedullary nails.

Not a total joint

22. The total hip has been a great success because it tends to be pain-free, but the hip is a weight-bearing joint; it was felt that the elbow, being a non-weight-bearing joint, would

do well without total joint replacement, and such has proved to be the case in most instances. We did one total elbow - using the above mentioned prosthesis plus a high density polyethylene insert in the semilunar notch. That patient has actually had more problems (due to instability) than those in which only the humeral side of the joint was replaced. Of course, total elbow joint replacement is necessary in those who have extreme trauma - who have little humerus or ulna left with which to re-build a joint.

Range of motion

23. Of our case series of eighteen patients, fourteen have excellent range of motion, averaging ninety degrees of flexion and extension, with full pronation and supination. Of those who were working prior to their injury or illness, most are back at their accustomed occupations. My favorite patient is our first one - an electrician, disabled for six years, when, a year after emplacement of the prosthesis went back to work as an electrician, which he has been again for the past nine years, whose range of motion in his previously ankylosed arm is only fifteen degrees less than that of his uninjured arm.

24. In our correspondence with our colleagues, most report very favorable ranges of motion.

25. However, we have had our problems with range of motion in a few cases. In experimenting with a new idea, one learns from the bad results as well as the good ones. One must accept all challenges, no matter how great, and draw conclusions from one's results. One must accept, in one's experimental series, absolutely the worst patients; in fact one must actively seek out the worst patients, as acid proof of one's ideas. And so we come to:

Problem areas

26. Four patients in our series have extremely poor to absent range of motion. One is a hemophiliac, aged 16 when operated on, who grew new bone about the prosthesis with remarkable rapidity. He has about 10 degrees of flexion-extension five years post surgery. Another is a man with extremely active rheumatoid arthritis, with two fused elbows, fused hips, a sed rate of 54 at the time of surgery. He also grew new bone, bridging the prosthesis, and has no range of motion. One, a Vietnam veteran, was a young man, hence an aggressive bone former, who also had severe neurological deficit of the injured arm, and hence was never able to carry out adequate post-operative physical therapy. His range of motion is 12 degrees. The fourth patient had ankylosis due to trauma, is two years post surgery, and his range of motion is apparently, according to Dr. Street, probably due to excessive scarring of the capsule, not to bone growth, and I believe a capsulectomy is planned for him. Because this prosthesis replaces so little bone, patients who are aggressive bone-formers, such as young people, or people with very active arthritic diseases, will grow new bone. This class of patient is thus not a candidate for the prosthesis. Another individual who is

obviously not a candidate is one who has had massive destruction of the distal humerus and proximal radius and ulna, as in a severe gunshot wound, where there is no bone to affix the prosthesis to, or for it to articulate with.

Candidates for the aforementioned prosthesis

27. All persons who have reached the age of bone maturity, who have elbow pathology requiring surgical intervention, (limited range of motion, pain with motion, etc.), who do not have a very active arthritic disease, such as active rheumatoid arthritis or hemophilia, who have not lost more than one inch of distal humeral bone, and who have an ulna with a semilunar notch, or enough ulna so a semilunar notch may be fashioned, or persons who have burned out rheumatoid arthritis or osteoarthritis in any stage of activity, are good candidates for the prosthesis.

Conclusions

28. a) The elbow is now, like the hip, repairable by prosthesis. b) The above-mentioned prosthesis is very effective in many types of elbow pathology. c) New prosthetic development for specialized situations is still necessary, and is underway.

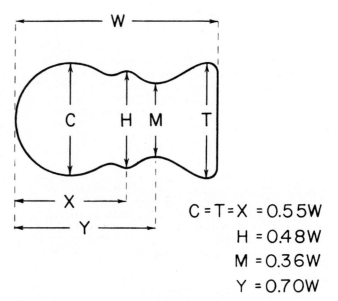

$$C = T = X = 0.55W$$
$$H = 0.48W$$
$$M = 0.36W$$
$$Y = 0.70W$$

Fig. 1:

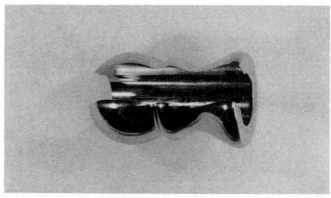

Fig. 2:

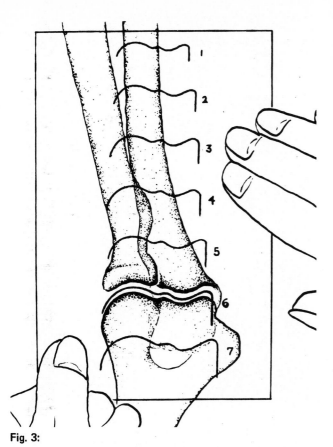

Fig. 3:

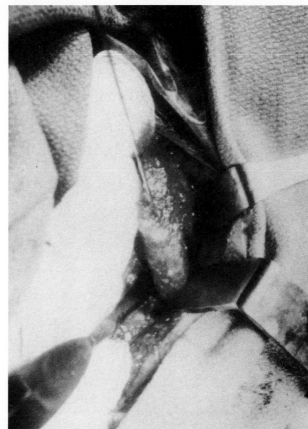

Fig. 4:

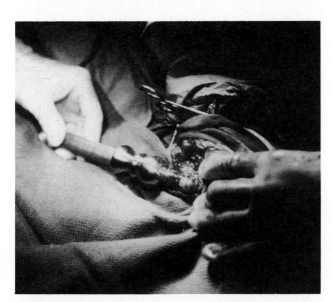

Fig. 5:

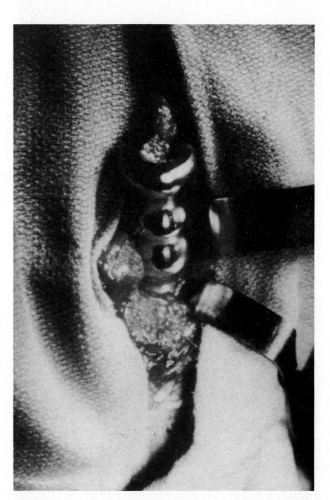

Fig. 6:

73

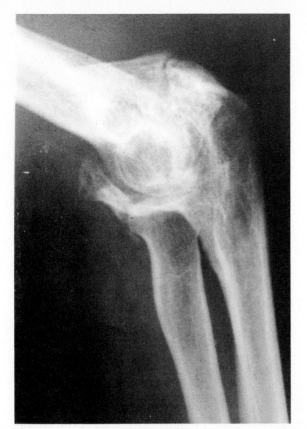
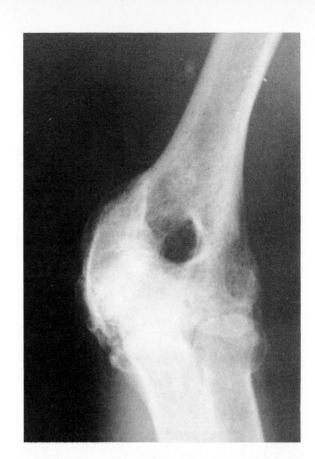

Fig. 7a:

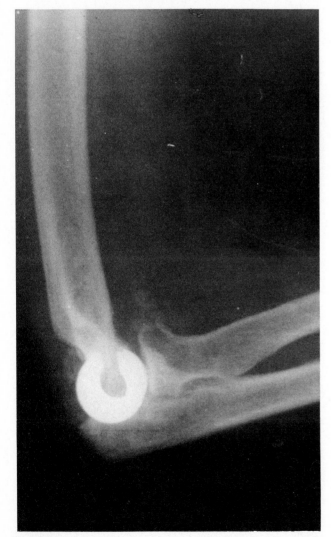
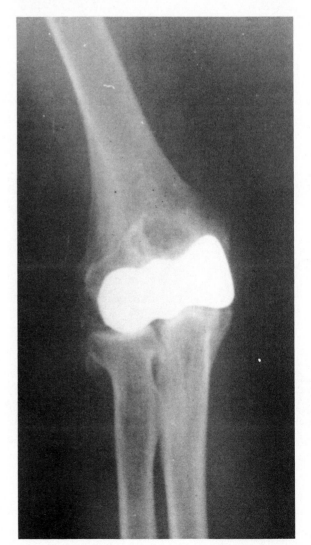

Fig. 7b:

74

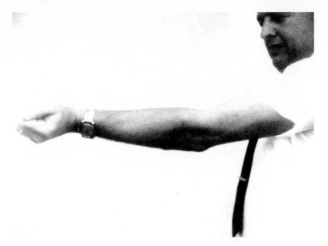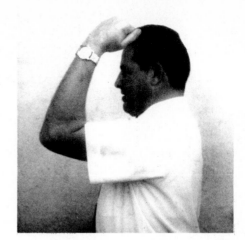

Fig. 7c:

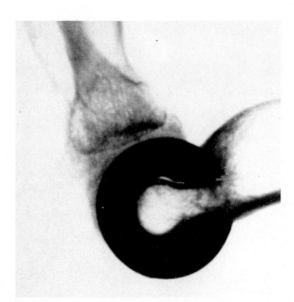

Fig. 8:

C160/77

NON-CONSTRAINED METAL TO PLASTIC TOTAL ELBOW ARTHROPLASTY IN RHEUMATOID ARTHRITIS

F.C. EWALD, MD, W.H. THOMAS, MD, C.B. SLEDGE, MD,
R.D. SCOTT, MD, and R. POSS, MD,
Harvard Medical School, Robert B. Brigham Hospital

SYNOPSIS   A non-constrained metal to plastic total elbow replacement has been implanted in 50 patients with rheumatoid arthritis. Maximum follow-up is two years nine months and minimum follow-up six months. There has been a significant increase in postoperative flexion ($\bar{x} = 135^\circ$ $p \ll .005$) and pronation ($\bar{x} = 71^\circ$ $p < .0025$) but no significant increase in postoperative extension or supination. Pain relief and functional improvement have been uniformly excellent based on a predetermined rating system (pre-op 36%, post-op 92%).

Three procedures have failed because of sepsis, previous fascial arthroplasty and persistent dislocation in unrecognized severe cubitus valgus. There has been no loosening of either component clinically or radiographically.

1.   INTRODUCTION

A metal to plastic elbow resurfacing prosthesis has been designed and developed in an effort to avoid problems seen with the single center metal hinge type of elbow replacement. These problems have been mainly loosening but triceps rupture and avascular necrosis have also been reported. (1,2,3)

2.   BIOMECHANICS

2.1   Elbow Motion
The elbow joint is not a rigid hinge mechanism and consists of three distinct articulations: ulnar-trochlear, radial-capitellar, and proximal radial-ulnar.

Elbow motion has been studied in cadavers (4) and in the frontal plane cubitus valgus of 10° changes to cubitus varus of 5° from full extension to full flexion. In addition, the forearm rotates about its longitudinal axis 5° internally and externally during flexion. The end of the humerus shows the trochlea and capitellum to run obliquely from lateral to medial starting with the extension surface and moving to the flexion surface. (5) This can cause a medial shift of the ulna on the humerus during flexion. Although it has been reported in cadavers that the elbow joint has a single center of rotation in the lateral plane, (4) two separate elbows in living patients were studied radiographically to determine the center of rotation, and the results showed a multi-axis in both patients. The center of rotation of the elbow remains controversial, but there is overwhelming evidence the elbow joint is not a simple hinge but a complex mechanism.

2.2   Forces and Testing
The joint reactive forces have been calculated for an arbitrary elbow position of 90° flexion in the sagittal plane and various weights placed in the hand. (6) This measurement includes the weight of the forearm and assumes the biceps, brachialis and brachioradialis muscles develop equal tension.

(Fig. 1) The joint reactive force (Fig. 2) is eight times the hand force and these numbers agree with our calculations and Walker's.(7) Using these forces the unit loading for the metal to plastic elbow prosthesis can be calculated. The measured surface area of metal to plastic contact for the non-constrained elbow prosthesis is 0.82 square inches, and the pounds per square inch is seen in figure 2. The unit loading is well below that calculated for the Charnley and the Charnley-Mueller total hip prosthesis. However, the metal to plastic interface has been studied by Walker in an elbow simulator that developed 50 lb. force in phase I through an arc of 45° and was lubricated with distilled water. The depth of penetration or wear of the metal into the plastic component was measured per million cycles in the simulator.

2.3   Radial Head
The biomechanical importance of the radial head in the normal elbow has been studied by Walker. (8) He examined six fresh intact elbows by recording a longitudinal force deflection curve. It is apparent from this work that up to 10 lb. longitudinal force applied along the forearm is transmitted via the interosseous membrane to the ulna-trochlear joint. At forces greater than ten lb., two-thirds of the force is transmitted through the radial-capitellar articulation. In patients with rheumatoid arthritis, the joints above and below the elbow are most often severely involved, and it is unlikely these patients would be capable of developing high longitudinal forces along the forearm. Therefore, in the rheumatoid patient the radial-capitellar and the proximal radial-ulnar joints are handled by radial head resection with the non-constrained prosthesis. However, in the case of a post-traumatic elbow where only one joint is involved, we are dealing with otherwise normal individuals capable of producing large forces during activities of daily living. For these patients, a polyethylene radial head replacement has been designed along with a metal ulnar fixation stem into which the

polyethylene ulnar component is press fitted. The lateral proximal edge of the metal stem provides for replacement of the proximal radial ulnar joint along with the polyethylene radial head prosthesis.

3.   PROSTHETIC DESIGN

The articular surfaces of the non-constrained elbow prosthesis were developed by carrying an average sized distal humeral model through a functional range of motion in a cooling bath of dental base plate wax.   The wax impression was then used as the surface configuration for the ulnar component.

Extensive radiographic measurements provided the proper size, attitude and angles for the fixation plug of the polyethylene ulnar component and the fixation stem of the metal humeral component.

The prosthesis is made for right and left elbows with two sizes for the polyethylene ulnar component and four variations of humeral fixation stem valgus (5^0, 10^0, 15^0, 20^0).   (Fig. 3)

4.   OPERATIVE TECHNIQUE

4.1   Introduction

Since the prosthetic components are not linked together, and the articulation is non-constrained, the soft tissues are very important to maintain stability and prevent dislocation.   The principles behind this type of arthroplasty is to allow the compressive joint reactive forces (sagittal plane forces) to be applied perpendicular to the tangent of the articular surface and rotational torque and oblique stress be absorbed by the soft tissues (capsule, ligaments and muscles) before being transmitted to the bone-cement interface.   The operative technique therefore demands careful preservation and anatomic restoration of the soft tissues.

The patient is placed in the lateral position and the joint approached posteromedially after careful dissection of the ulnar nerve.   The triceps tendon is taken down at the musculotendinous junction in a 'V' shaped incision with the base on the olecranon.   The joint capsule is cleaned of soft tissue on three sides, and the joint is entered in a 'T' shaped capsular incision following the borders of the trochlear notch of the ulna.   The corners of the capsular incision are marked for later repair.   The key to adequate exposure is dissection of the capsule and extensor and flexor tendons out to the origins of the medial and lateral capsular collateral ligaments near the tip of the medial and lateral epicondyles.

Only a small amount of bone is resected from the ulna and humerus to insert the components because they are essentially surface replacements. Most of the bone removal is for the humeral and ulnar fixation stems.   Both the metal and plastic components have three point fixation; the humeral component caps the remnants of the trochlea and capitellum and has a medullary stem, and the ulnar component has two fixation runners for the two sides of the trochlear notch of the ulna with a medullary stem as well.   Insertion and alignment of the components is described elsewhere.   (9)   The capsular and collateral ligaments are carefully re-approximated with permanent suture so the prosthesis will not dislocate or subluxate and so the elbow will have a satisfactory range of motion.   The triceps tendon is sutured to its original bed.

4.2   Postoperative Regimen

The postoperative physical therapy programme is extremely important and progressive active-assistive range of motion exercises are started twice daily on the third postoperative day.   The elbow is held in a posterior extension splint at night and a sling at 90^0 during the day.   At ten days postoperative, activities of daily living exercises are started with the elbow held at the side.   Two weeks postoperative, the patient is discharged on a home physical therapy programme of exercises, sling during the day and splint at night for an additional two weeks.   One month postoperative, the sling and night splint are discarded, but the patient is cautioned not to reach out from the side to pick up objects for an additional two weeks.   Six weeks postoperative when the capsular healing is complete, normal activities of daily living may be resumed.   Return to heavy labor or sports such as tennis are not recommended.

5.   CLINICAL TRIALS AND RESULTS

5.1   Patients

Fifty elbows have been implanted in 46 patients all with well documented rheumatoid arthritis. Thirty-eight are female and eight are male, and the average age is 60.   The first procedure in this series was performed on July 22, 1974 and the last on September 9, 1976.   Maximum follow-up is two years and nine months, minimum follow-up six months with a median of one and a half years.

5.2   Results

The clinical results have been assessed in a number of ways, one of which is a prospective elbow evaluation form (Fig. 4) that is based on 100 points for a normal elbow.   Fifty-percent is allotted for pain, 30% for function, 10% for motion, and 10% for deformity.   The average pre-op rating was 36 and the average post-op rating taken two or more months postoperative has been 92.   This rating average is under continuous review and there has been no change during the follow-up period noted above.

Pre- and postoperative elbow motion is seen in figure 5 and there has been a significant increase in average postoperative flexion and pronation, but the small increases seen in extension and supination are not statistically significant.

5.3   Complications

A list of complications is seen in figure 6.   The one permanent ulnar nerve palsy occurred in a patient with a peripheral rheumatoid neuropathy and an atrophic nerve.   The transient ulnar nerve palsy was thought to be due to thermal injury from curing methacrylate.   The ulnar nerve is not routinely transposed anteriorly.

One patient developed deep Peptococcus sepsis after failure of the skin incision to heal.   The olecranon process protruded posteriorly because the plastic component was placed into a large bony defect created by a giant rheumatoid cyst. This early case prompted design of an optional thick plastic ulnar component.   (Fig. 3)

Two patients dislocated postoperatively and were easily reduced and have been stable for over one year.   One of the patients was reaching out and lifting a five pound handbag one week post-operative when the elbow dislocated, and the other dislocated for unknown reasons.

Another patient early in this series was

completely unstable in extension postoperative but had a previous failed fascial arthroplasty. At the time of surgery there were no ligaments or capsule to repair, and this elbow was eventually converted to a Pritchard-Walker 'loose' hinge arthroplasty.

The two biggest problems in this series were elbows that tracked poorly at the time of surgery and seemed to dislocate in a rotatory manner with the lateral soft tissues appearing very tight. Both of these elbows were never located post-operative and were found dislocated in the recovery room. After retrospective examination of previous x-rays, true A-P views of the distal humerus were found. This revealed cubitus valgus of 32° and 27° in both dislocated elbows. Clinical measurement of cubitus valgus in an elbow with a 20° to 30° flexion deformity is difficult and inaccurate. Likewise, most A-P x-rays of an elbow with a flexion deformity are oblique views. In a retrospective review of the x-rays of thirty preoperative cases, only half had true A-P views of the distal humerus. The cubitus valgus ranged from 5° to 32° in those able to be measured, and eight of the fifteen x-rays measured showed cubitus valgus greater than fifteen degrees. This probably indicates that the rheumatoid elbow can go into excessive valgus as the rheumatoid knee, but it is far more difficult to measure preoperatively. The reasons for the two dislocations with severe cubitus valgus became clear. Five degree valgus fixation stems for the humeral component were used in these elbows which had true valgus of 27° and 32°. This resulted in the lateral structures being too tight, the medial side of the joint too loose, and inherent instability with rotatory dislocation. These cases prompted the design of four different valgus stem angles. (Fig. 3) One of these cases was re-operated, a 15° valgus stem implanted, and this elbow has remained stable for the year following revision. The other patient could not be re-operated for one year due to a heart attack and skin problems and could not be surgically salvaged after that period of time.

In summary, the complications have resulted in three absolute failures. The first failure was due to deep sepsis, the second to an inappropriate indication (failed fascial arthroplasty), and the third to a technical problem (severe unrecognized cubitus valgus).

5.4   Contraindications
This experience has led to the following contraindications to the procedure:
1. Previous sepsis.
2. Previous fascial arthroplasty
3. Excessive loss of bone, as in giant rheumatoid cysts
4. Deficient trochlear notch of the ulnar
5. Post-traumatic or osteoarthritis
6. Previous hinge type arthroplasty

However, the newly designed radial head replacement and metal ulnar fixation stem described in the section on radial head may remove catagories 3, 4, and 5 from the contraindications list above.

6.   ADVANTAGES AND DISADVANTAGES

The main advantage of this arthroplasty is that there has been no documented loosening of either the metal or plastic component and no evidence of avascular necrosis to date. The main disadvantage is that there has not been a statisti-cally significant gain in postoperative extension. (Fig. 5)

REFERENCES

1. Souter, W. A. 'Arthroplasty of the Elbow', Ortho. Clin. N. Amer., 4:395-413, (April) 1973.

2. Dee, R. 'Total Replacement Arthroplasty of the Elbow for Rheumatoid Arthritis', Journal of Bone and Joint Surgery, 54B:88-95, (Feb) 1972.

3. Ewald, F. C. 'Total Elbow Replacement', Ortho. Clin. N. Amer., 6:685-696, (July) 1975.

4. Morrey, B. F. and Chao, E. Y. 'Passive Motion of the Elbow Joint. A Biomechanical Analysis', Journal of Bone and Joint Surgery, 58A:501-508, (June) 1976.

5. Barnett, C. H., Davies, D. V. and Mac Conaill, M. A. Synovial Joints, Springfield, Ill., C. C. Thomas, 1961.

6. Asher, M..A. and Zilber, S. 'Biomechanics of the Elbow and Forearm', A.A.O.S. Post-graduate Course in Elbow, Wrist and Forearm, Kansas City, Mo. (Oct. 13) 1973.

7. Walker, P. S. 'Forces in Joints', Human Joints and Their Artificial Replacements, Ch. 2, C. C. Thomas, Springfield, Ill. In press.

8. Walker, P. S. 'Laxity, Flexibility, and Stability', Human Joints and Their Artificial Replacements, Ch. 4, C. C. Thomas, Springfield, Ill. In press.

9. Ewald, F. C. 'Operative Technique, Non-Constrained Metal to Plastic Total Elbow Arthroplasty', Robert B. Brigham Hospital, Boston, Mass.

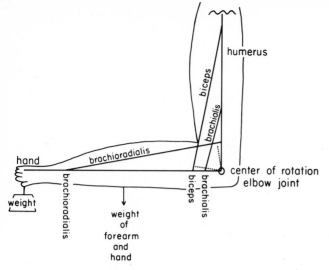

Fig. 1: Calculation of elbow joint reactive force

Activity	Joint Reactive Force - Lb.	P.S.I. Metal to Plastic T.E.R.
Lifting qt. of milk - 2 lb.	16	19
Lifting 1/2 gal. of milk - 4 lb.	32	39
Lifting 50 lb. weight - one hand	402	490

Fig. 2: Joint reactive force in normal and prosthetic elbow

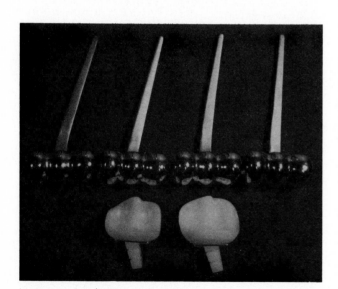

Fig. 3: Metal to plastic non-constrained total elbow prosthesis

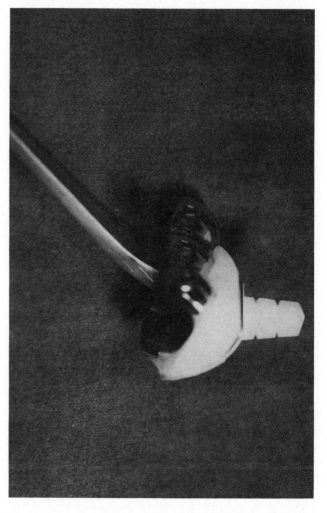

© IMechE 1977

80

ELBOW EVALUATION FORM

Name				Diag.
Hosp. #				Operation
Date of exam.				Surgeon
Date of surg.				R or L

Pain

None or ignores	50
Slight, occasional pain meds	45
Moderate, takes daily pain meds	35
Moderate, rest and/or night pain	15
Severe, disabled	0

Function

No limitations	30
Slight, no restriction of A.D.L.	25
Unable to lift heavy objects ($> 10\#$)	20
Moderate restriction of A.D.L.	10
Unable to comb hair or touch head	5
Unable to feed self	0

Motion

Flexion $> 130^{\circ}$	10
Flexion $110-130^{\circ}$	5
Flexion $90-110^{\circ}$	2
Flexion $< 90^{\circ}$	0

Deformity

P. F. C. $< 15^{\circ}$	5
P. F. C. $15^{\circ} - 30^{\circ}$	2
P. F. C. $> 30^{\circ}$	0

Valgus $0 - 10^{\circ}$	5
Cubitus varus $0 - 5^{\circ}$	2
Cubitus varus $> 5^{\circ}$	0

Patient Total

Pronation
Supination

Flexion
Extension

Fig. 4: Elbow evaluation form

ELBOW MOTION

	Flexion	Ext.	Pronation	Sup.
Pre-op	122±16	(-)34±15	53±25	54±24
Post-op	135±11	(-)29±14	71±17	62±24
P value	$< .0005$	$< .15$	$< .0025$	$< .10$

Fig. 5: Pre-and post-operative elbow motion

COMPLICATIONS

Ulnar nerve palsy	
Transient	1
Permanent	1
New bone formation	1
Sepsis	
Superficial	1
Deep	1
Dislocation, single event	2
Unstable in extension	1
(previous fascial arthro.)	
Never located post-op	2

Fig. 6: Complications

C161/77

TOTAL ELBOW REPLACEMENT WITH A HINGE AND A NON-BLOCKED SYSTEM

E. ENGELBRECHT, H.W. BUCHHOLZ, J. RÖTTGER, A. SIEGEL
Endo-Klinik, Hamburg, West Germany

SYNOPSIS   Five years' experience with 62 alloarthroplastic operations on the elbow joint
are reported. Painful, unstable and ankylosed joints are successfully treated by replacement with a hinge prosthesis. Due to a limited loading capacity the indications for this
prosthesis are still restricted. The main causes for complications are deep infection,
mechanical loosening and a false operative technique. Our own experiences have led to
changes in construction and hence to significant improvements of the design. For two
years we have experimented with a non-blocked type of prosthesis, the so-called
'rolling prosthesis', but in spite of encouraging initial results further development
is necessary.

1.   Special problems in the treatment of
severely unstable or ankylosed elbow joints
in patients with rheumatoid arthritis have
evoked the desire to transfer the principles
of alloarthroplastic replacement of the hip
and knee joint to the elbow joint.
The first hinge prosthesis constructed in
1970-71 was based on the following principles:
1) Low-Friction Arthroplasty (LFA)
2) Polyethylene for the humeral component
in order
a) to gain a shock-absorbing effect and
b) to make a first approach towards an iso-
elastic prosthesis and
3) a most economical joint resection and
optimal covering of the implant with body-
own tissue structures.

2.   Zippel was the first who designed a
mono-blocked hinge prosthesis according to
these principles. Due to problems in the
operative technique a model made of two parts
was designed shortly thereafter. Therefore,
two different modifications were in use:
The BME (Biomechanical Endoprosthesis) design
by Zippel and the design 'St.Georg' differing
in the ulnar component and the closing
mechanism.

3.   The hinge prosthesis, design 'St.Georg',
had a humeral part of polyethylene and an
ulnar part of metal. Both components were
joined by a running axis which was inserted
laterally. The axis was fixed to the ulnar
part with a screw. Accordant with the physiological axis of rotation within the elbow
joint the prosthetic turning point was set
ventrally. The range of movement of the hinge
corresponded with the range of movement of
the natural joint. The design was available
of two different sizes.

4.   Experiences have shown that several
disadvantageous criteria of the prosthesis
had to be altered. Polyethylene as a material
for the humeral part of the prosthesis was

no longer used, since especially in active
and strong patients the plastic material did
not in any case meet the requirements of permanent loading conditions, a fact, resulting
in mechanical loosening. For the sake of
stability the humeral component within the
supra-epicondylar region was given a rather
heavy shape which sometimes either required
a too extensive bone resection or a reduction in size of the polyethylene part in
smaller joints. A lateral insertion of the
running axis through a drill hole in the
radial epicondyle occasionally resulted in
less stability of the epicondylar bone with
danger of bone fracture.

5.   For this reason we now use a hinged
prosthesis - corresponding to the first
design - but with two metal components and
a polyethylene bearing in the proximal part
maintaining the principles of LFA with
decisive improvement of prosthetic stability (Fig. 1). The shape of the supra-epicondylar part was altered in order to keep
the necessary bone resection within small
dimensions. A modified closing mechanism
makes drill holes in the epicondylar bone
useless. The axis within the polyethylene
bearing is inserted via a slit in the ulnar
part and firmly fixed with a screw. The
range of movement corresponds to the physiological movability of the joint.

6.   As is the case with the knee joint the
hinge prosthesis of the elbow does not
correspond to the physiological movability.
In cases of intramedullary fixation the
dimensions of the implant must be kept
small due to anatomical conditions resulting in a relatively small contact area
between implant and bone. Due to the long
levers of the upper arm and the lower arm
extreme forces are acting on the bone causing increase in bone resorption and possibly loosening of the implant. A restriction
to proper function of the shoulder joint

may, for example, intensify the lever action of the lower arm on the humeral prosthetic component just as a restricted rotatory motion of the lower arm may intensify the lever action on the ulnar prosthetic component. These problems finally led to the conclusion that a non-blocked prosthesis should be given a special shape in order to transmit forces acting on the joint to the surrounding soft tissues.

6.   The first design, a so-called 'rolling prosthesis', has been clinically used since the middle of 1974 (2, 4, 9). This prosthesis consists of two non-blocked parts with a range of movement of O-145 degrees. The humeral component replacing the trochlea is made of polyethylene and formed like a bobbin. A metallic axis equiped with two stems, one on each side, provides a firm fixation within the supra-epicondylar region where we may expect stable cortical bone. This method of fixation guarantees more safety against rotatory forces. The ulnar component resembles the olecranon in shape; the prosthetic stem slightly bent towards ventral is anchored in the medullary canal of the ulna. The two running surfaces of the prosthesis coincide in shape, but when tilting they make way for each other and transmit forces to the surrounding soft tissues (Fig. 2). In previous operative techniques the head of the radius was removed but now we are of the opinion that it should be preserved with regard to better joint stability. We therefore try - if possible - to preserve both the capitulum humeri and the head of the radius and perform a meticulous synovectomy in cases of rheumatoid arthritis; osteophyts are removed and the bone made smooth.
We hope that further modifications of the design and a simultaneous replacement of the capitulum humeri and the head of the radius will not only improve stability but also enable both prosthetic components to make way for each other in the process of motion. An intact or tightenable ligamentous apparatus of the joint is mandatory for the use of a non-blocked prosthesis.

Operative technique

7.   Surgery is performed with a tourniquet and if possible with the patient prone and the arm hanging down. If a supine position of the patient is inevitable the extremity is positioned on an arm-table or on a cushion.
Different approaches to the joint have been used. A curved incision beginning dorsally and leading convexly over the joint has the advantage of less soft tissues being mobilized. Through this approach the triceps tendon was seperated either subperiostially, about 1 cm proximal to the olecranon or by a transversal incision of the tendon. However, this approach requires careful and reserved after-treatment with inherent danger of insufficiency of the triceps tendon; therefore this approach is no longer chosen. We now approach the joint through an ulnar convexo-dorsal skin incision in the longitudinal direction. The tendon of the triceps muscle is divided with a V-shape incision at the transition zone of tendon and muscle.

On the insertion of the hinge prosthesis the collateral ligaments can be resected tangentially to the epicondyles without fear of disadvantages. Advantageous is the good view we gain of the joint, especially when a complete synovectomy is performed routinely in cases of rheumatoid arthritis. The fascia of the forearm is dissected medially and laterally from the olecranon down to the plane of the head of the radius in the longitudinal direction, and the soft tissue is carefully stripped from the ulna. Hitherto we used to remove the head of the radius. An intraepicondylar block corresponding to the width of the prosthesis is sawn out, and the medullary canal of the humerus is prepared for insertion of the humeral part of the prosthesis. The articulating surface of the olecranon and some portion of the proc.coronoides are removed. The medullary cavity of the ulna is next prepared and the ulnar component inserted. During a test run the surgeon has to decide whether a further resection either on the ulna or on the humerus is necessary. Any present flexion contraction may be corrected in this way (Fig. 3).
After release of tourniquet both components are cemented in place with Refobacin-Palacos ^{R}. Any cement surplus must be carefully removed in order to avoid wear. After insertion of the axis into the ulnar part the blocking screw is inserted and plugged with Palacos bone cement.
After joint drainage both ends of the triceps tendon are adapted with interrupted Certofil stitches followed by subcutaneous drainage. The skin is closed with a monophile suture. The joint is carefully covered with soft pads, and a removable plaster splint is applied holding the upper arm in 45° abduction to the longitudinal axis of the body. The operative procedure for the insertion of a 'rolling prosthesis' differs only in some points. Maintenance of collateral ligaments is mandatory. The intraepicondylar block is sawn out and the medullary canal of the humerus opened medially and laterally corresponding to the anchoring stems of the humeral component leaving the fossa olecrani intact. The capitulum humeri and the head of the radius are maintained. Irregularities should only be smoothed and exophytes removed as long as they restrict rotation. In cases of rheumatoid arthritis a resection of the distal portion of the ulna is performed, if necessary, in order to improve rotational movement.

Postoperative treatment

8.   The arm is placed in an upright position using a plaster splint and the patient is asked to elevate the arm above the head as frequently as possible. Isometric muscle training and measures against swelling are initiated immediately after surgery by the physiotherapist. Active exercises are instituted as soon as postoperative pain subsides, between the 4th and 6th day. For this purpose only the plaster splint is removed, but otherwise it should be in place for 8 to 14 days. Thereafter the predominating active exercises are slowly but continually increased. Preventive measures against thrombosis are not needed when the patient is mobilized one day after surgery.

Results

9.   In the period 1971 to 1976, 64 elbow joint prostheses have been inserted in a total of 53 patients. In 9 cases a prosthesis was inserted on both sides, in 44 cases on one side. The average age was 56 years (22-84 years). 2/3 (two third) of the patients were female.
The results of our follow-up investigations are related to 49 patients (80 per cent) followed over an average period of 18 months (minimum 4 months, maximum 48 months).

9.   Rheumatoid arthritis and post-traumatic arthrosis are the main indications for the hinged elbow joint prosthesis. It is especially indicated in cases of rheumatoid arthritis with very painful and severely unstable or ankylosed joints as well as in cases of post-traumatic arthrosis with restriction of movement and almost stiff and very painful joints. Robust and very active or physically hard-working patients are not suited for elbow joint replacement (Table 1).

10.   From our own experiences we have drawn the conclusion that the indication for an unblocked prosthesis is restricted to those with a widely intact ligamentous apparatus. We hope that in the near future the allo-arthroplasty of the elbow joint can be extended on cases where the joint is exposed to more physical activity. The results given are not classified according to various types of prostheses, as in this respect no differences have been observed.

11. Results of joint function.

Experiences have shown that with a prosthetic replacement of the elbow joint we not only maintain the present function of the joint but also improve joint movability. Ankylosed joints over many years can be remobilized successfully. Remarkable differences between rheumtaoid arthritis and post-traumatic arthrosis regarding improvement of rotatory motion may be explained by the fact that in cases of rheumatoid arthritis, the wrist is involved as well. Functional improvement is equally distributed to extension, flexion, internal and external rotation. To date no significant differences have been observed. In 80 per cent of the cases we found a residual extension deficiency of 10 degrees (0°-40°) on the average.

12. Results concerning pain.

Although 30 per cent of the followed patients with ankylosis had been painfree preoperatively, the postoperative percentage raised to 67 per cent after the implantation of a total prosthesis. The most frequent remaining pain conditions may be related to complications demanding reoperation. The predominant pain conditions are scar pain and sensitivity to weather changes. Poor results may be referred to loosening of the implant or infections.

Complications (Table 2)

13.   Due to the modified shape of the hinged prosthesis and the closing mechanism intraoperative fractures on the epicondylar bone (4 cases) should no longer occur. Insufficiency of the triceps tendon was only observed 4 times after subperiosteal separation or transversal division of the triceps tendon proximal to its insertion at the olecranon. We therefore have altered our operative technique so that now the V-shaped division of the triceps tendon is used exclusively.
In one case Sudeck's disease was observed but healed completely under conservative medical treatment.
Patients with postoperative actopic bone formation (2 cases) have not been operated on. Their joint function was poor with residual pain conditions.
Loosening of the ulnar part was due to a false operative technique with perforation of the cortex or to an insufficient amount of bone cement. In one case recurrent synovitis may possibly have caused loosening. Exchange of ulnar component was successfully performed in two cases.
Loosening of the humeral component of the polyethylene design was only observed within the supra-epicondylar area. We are of the opinion that this must be referred to inadequate rigidity of polyethylene. In all four cases the patients were very active and strong. This observation was the reason for giving up utilizing the polyethylene model and to develop the metal prosthesis according to the LFA principle. The change from the polyethylene model to a metal model led to good and satisfactory results.
We had two cases with deep infection. Reoperation was performed with Refobacin-Palacos ^{R} bone cement and an additional dosage of Refobacin (gentamicin) and failed in one case. The prosthesis had to be removed and the final result is poor. The joint is unstable and the patient has to wear an external splint apparatus. The second infected case was not evaluated since the patient died two months after surgery because of renal insufficiency.
In one case where a 'rolling prosthesis' was inserted loosening of the humeral part was observed. This was due to a false indication for this design. In this case of rheumatoid arthritis with severe instability of the joint we immobilized the joint and applied a fixateur extern for some weeks postoperatively, but the joint remained unstable. Permanent instability of the collateral ligaments with recurrent joint dislocations are likely to have caused loosening of the humeral part. The prosthesis was removed and a hinge prosthesis inserted.
After remobilizing an ankylosed joint in a case of rheumatoid arthritis by means of a 'rolling prosthesis', dislocation was observed due to lateral instability. We applied a fixateur extern for a period of some weeks, and the result was satisfactory; the joint was painfree, though functional movement was restricted (extension/flexion 60°/130°, rotation 90°).

The total rate of severe complications of 20 per cent reflects lack of experiences at the beginning. Elbow joint replacement is still under development. Corrective measures will surely reduce the high rate of complications below 5 per cent. Further improvements on the design and in the operative technique and a very strict indication will definitely lower the rate of failure.

Discussion

14.   Five years of experiences with 62 alloarthroplastic operations have enlarged our knowledge regarding design, scope and operative technique for the total elbow joint replacement and given impulses to further development.
The low number of operations is due to the following criteria: non-weight-bearing joints of the upper extremity do not often require operative measures. The good results achieved with synovectomy and resection arthroplasty still offer an alternative. Difficulties in designing a suitable and more generally applicable implant will also in the near future still confine the number of alloarthroplastic operations on the elbow joint.

15.   Experiences over 5 years have enabled us to make clear statements about our clinical results. The hinge prosthesis does not only provide immediate stability of the joint but also painfree joint movability. The preoperative movability of the joint will be maintained or improved. Ankylosed joints of many years are successfully remobilized.

16.   Some criteria of construction of our first design have proved disadvantageous and required further development. The polyethylene design did not guarantee sufficient stability and the shape of the implant did not allow economical resection of bone. According to our present experiences only the metal design meets with the demands of stability and economical resection. The principles of LFA must be maintained in any case in order to avoid metallosis which sometimes presents itself years after surgery. Furthermore, the interposition of polyethylene guarantees low friction and a shock-absorbing effect. Forces acting on the anchoring parts are approximately 2-3 times the forces acting on the hip joint, which must be related to the long levers of the upper and lower arm (1).
One must consider that rotational forces act upon the anchorage of the humeral part of the prosthesis and that shear forces, developing in the process of flexion and extension act on the anchorage of both components of the prosthesis. Therefore, the routine resection of the head of the radius is not advisable because we lose a stabilizing component. There is every reason to believe that under extreme strain conditions bone reacts with resorption at the junction of bone and bone cement; i.e. that mechanical loosening of the hinged prosthesis of the elbow joint may occur more often than in other joints.

17.   In order to avoid this complication a design should be feasible where forces are transmitted to long prosthetic stems and where apart from polyethylene an additional absorbing factor is inserted into the hinge. But both possibilities are limited by the demand for small dimensions. Another possible energy absorbing design is the non-blocked gliding prosthesis. The components running against oneanother should be designed that way that withdrawing movements are possible and that forces can be transmitted to the surrounding tissues. A first approach in this respect is our 'rolling prosthesis'.
First clinical experiences are encouraging but the range of indication is limited. Further development is based on the improvement of shape and an additional joint stabilizing effect by replacing the capitulum humeri and radi. Whether the range of application may be extended so far, that in future only the 'rolling prosthesis' is used, is still doubted. Probably two types of implants will be used as we have for the knee joint.
At present the hinged prosthesis of the elbow joint may be regarded as an effective method in treating unstable or ankylosed joints successfully. A careful indication is required and should be restricted to old patients and patients suffering from rheumatoid arthritis where no extreme physical activity is expected. (5, 6, 7, 8) With a further development of our unblocked prosthesis we see a chance of extending the range of indication in future.

REFERENCES

1. BOUWER S.   Indications and Results of elbow prosthesis. Congres annuel de la societé belge de chirurgie orthopedique et de traumatologie, Gent, May 1975.

2. BURROUGH S.J.   The design of an elbow prosthesis. Eng.Med.2,64(1973)

3. ENGELBRECHT E. and ZIPPEL J.   Totale Ellengelenksendoprothese Modell 'St.Georg'. Chirurg 46,232,490(1975

4. ENGELBRECHT E.   A new elbow replacement Acta orthop.belg.41,484(1975)

5. DEE R.   Total replacement arthroplasty of the elbow for rheumatoid arthritis. J.Bone Jt.Surg.54 B,88(1972

6. DEE R.   Total prosthesis of the elbow. Acta orthop.belg.41,477(1975)

7. GSCHWEND N., SCHEIER H. and BÄHLER A. GSB-Ellbogen-Endoprothese. Arch.orthop. Unfall-Chir.73,316(1972)

8. GSCHWEND N.   Our experience of elbow arthroplasty with the GSB Prosthesis. Acta orthop.belg.41,470(1975)

9. STEEVENS P.S. and STREET D.M.   The use of the Stevens-Street elbow prosthesis. Acta orthop.belg.41,447(1975)

TABLE I

DESIGN	DIAGNOSIS	
ST. GEORG - POLYETHYLENE MODIFICATION (N = 45) BME - MODEL (N = 5)	RHEUMATOID ARTHRITIS	32
	RHEUMATOID ANKYLOSIS	9
	POSTTR. ARTHROSIS	3
	POSTTR. ANKYLOSIS	6
ST. GEORG - METAL MODIFICATION (LOW FRICTION) (N = 7)	RHEUMATOID ARTHRITIS	5
	POSTTR. ARTHROSIS	1
	POSTTR. ANKYLOSIS	1
NON-BLOCKED-SYSTEM "ROLLING-PROSTHESIS" (N = 7)	RHEUMATOID ARTHRITIS	4
	RHEUMATOID ANKYLOSIS	1
	POSTTR. ARTHROSIS	1
	IDIOPATHIC ARTHROSIS	1
TOTAL		64

TABLE II

DESIGN	COMPLICATION	CAUSE	CORRECTIVE TREATMENT	FINAL RESULTS		
				good	fair	poor
ST. GEORG-POLYETHYLENE MODIFICATION	LOOSENING OF THE ULNARY COMPONENT 4	PERFORATION OF THE CORTEX INSUFFICIENT CEMENTING	EXCHANGING 2	2	2	-
	LOOSENING OF THE HUMERAL COMPONENT 4	INSUFFICIENT STABILITY OF HDP	CONVERSION OF DESIGN 4	2	1	1
	LOOSENING OF BOTH COMPONENTS 2	DEEP INFECTION	REMOVAL 1 PAT.✠ 1	- -	- -	1 1
NON-BLOCKED SYSTEM	LOOSENING OF THE HUMERAL COMPONENT 1	REMAINING INSTABILITY	CONVERSION OF DESIGN 1	1	-	-
	POST.-OPERATIVE DISLOCATION 1	LACK OF STABILITY AFTER REMOBILISATION OF AN ANKYLOSIS	STABILISATION BY FIXATEUR EXTERN	1	-	-

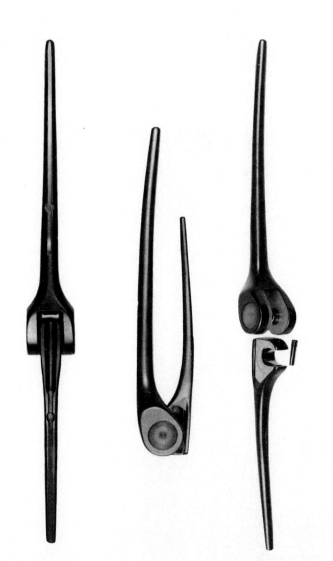

Fig. 1: A hinge prosthesis design 'St. Georg' — metal modification

Fig. 2: Left: first design of the non-blocked 'rolling prothesis'
Right: a design for further development

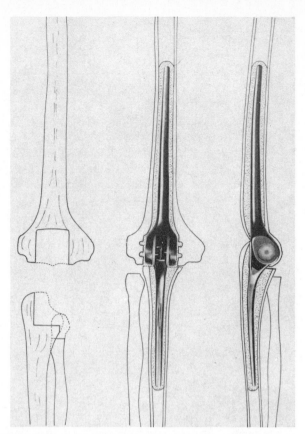

Fig. 3: Joint resection for replacement with a hinged prosthesis

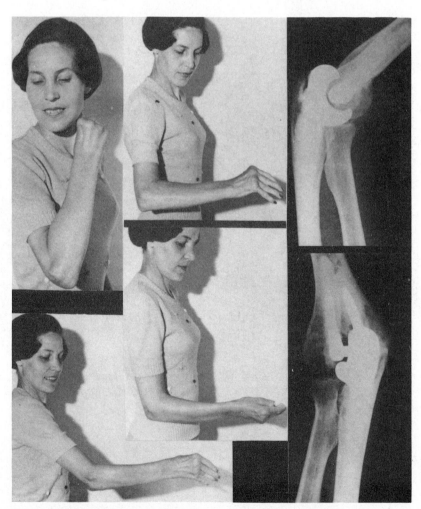

Fig. 4: Female, 36, rheumatoid arthritis, 18 months after implantation of a 'rolling prosthesis'. Painfree joint. Improvement of function: Extension/flexion 40° rotation 50°

FIVE YEARS' EXPERIENCE WITH TOTAL REPLACEMENT OF THE ELBOW

R. DEE, FRCS, PhD
Dept. of Orthopaedic Surgery,
State University of New York at Stony Brook,
Stony Brook, New York 11794, USA

SYNOPSIS   A long term follow-up of 40 elbow arthroplasties using Dee hinge is reported. They were 32 female and 6 male, average age 52. Seventeen left arthroplasties and nineteen right arthroplasties and two bilateral arthroplasties were in the series. Thirty-five patients had rheumatoid arthritis and the remainder had previous elbow trauma. Results show 21 arthroplasties were good but 12 elbows were poor and 7 were considered fair. Complications were infrequent and not serious with the exception of the problem of loosening. There were two cases of serious infection and in one case the joint was removed. There were some superficial skin necroses in 4 cases. There were 3 cases of hematomata. There were 5 cases of ulna nerve irritability but no severe neuro-vascular complications. There were 11 loose joints in the series and the majority of these cases occurred more than two years from surgery. Eight of these have gross thinning of the cortex and severe symptoms and have been revised and the other 3 at this time do not have sufficient indication to require removal of the hinge. Revision has been found to be difficult. Different methods have been tried with a varying degree of success to stabilize elbow after removal of the loose hinge. The best solution has been found by using a specially designed semi-constrained prosthesis which is described in detail. The errors of design in the elbow hinge which render this joint now obsolete are discussed. Some reasons for optimism that the new semi-constrained metal/plastic joint with a snap fit mechanism may be more durable are given.

1.   I reported (Ref. 1) the results of artho-plasty using a prosthesis of my own design some five years ago. This was the first published account of a series of elbow replacements. The unusual feature of the new prosthesis was that it had specially curved medullary stems suitable for use with acrylic cement. The initial results were exceedingly successful and the time has come for a longer term assessment.

CLINICAL MATERIAL

2.   Forty arthoplasties were reviewed in a group of 32 females and 6 males, varying in age from 32 to 64 (average age, 52). There were 17 left elbow replacements and 19 right elbow re-placements; 2 patients had bilateral replacements. All the patients have a follow-up period varying from two to five years since operation.

Indications

3.   Thirty-five of the patients had rheumatoid arthritis and most of this group included patients with painful instability although there were six patients with ankylosis, three of whom had com-plete bony ankylosis prior to surgery. All the non-rheumatoid patients had had previous trauma to the elbow.

Assessment

4.   A patient with 90° or more of painfree move-ment in the useful arc was assessed as good;

45° to 90° of movement, painfree, in a useful arc was assessed as a fair result. Less than 45° of movement or significant pain or discharging sinus or some other complication put that patient into the category of poor.

RESULTS

5.   In this follow-up there were 21 artho-plasties still classified as good, 7 elbows were fair, and 12 elbows were considered poor.

Complications

6. Infection: There were two serious infections in the series. One elbow was treated unsuccess-fully for a deep infection commencing within one month of surgery. The joint was eventually re-moved, however the elbow continued to discharge and the patient was left with considerable insta-bility and the necessity to wear a supporting elbow splint permanently. Another patient had a superficial wound infection which completely responded to antibiotic therapy.

7. Other soft tissue problems: There was one ruptured triceps tendon occurring with avascular necrosis of the tip of the olecranon. This case has been reported in detail elsewhere (Ref. 2) and after modification of the technique, it was not a problem that occurred again. There were four cases of superficial necrosis of the margins of the wound showing that it is difficult

to handle large skin flaps on the extensor surface of the elbow, particularly in rheumatoid patients. Again, the surgery was modified so that a midline incision was used instead of a curving incision on the postero-lateral aspect of the joint. This considerably reduced the incidence of this complication. Similarly hematomata were a considerable problem occurring three times in the first ten cases. The use of subcutaneus drains as well as a deep drain soon eliminated this problem. There were five cases of transient ulnar nerve symptoms, but no paralysis. The nerve retained its irritability for several months following surgery, but eventually settled. Again, in the later cases instead of transplanting the nerve and leaving it subcutaneous, it was transplanted deep in a muscle bed and this abolished the incidence of the complication. At no time was there any major neurological or vascular complication of surgery.

8. Loosening: A major complication seen in this series was the grave problem of loosening. Three patients had obvious radiological loosening and one of these patients has radiological changes bilaterally in his arthoplasties. However, these patients have no severe pain at this time and therefore there are no plans for immediate revision. All three patients are rheumatoid patients with little demand on the upper limb and significantly none of them uses crutches. One of them surprisingly has no symptoms and is classified as a fair result. The other two are classified as poor results. Eight joints have been removed because of increasing pain and alarming erosion of the cortex (Fig. I). Five of these patients were rheumatoid. Of the total of 11 joint loosenings there are 5 identifiably loose ulna stems and 9 loose humeral stems.

9. Loosening occurred within one year in only two of these cases, and within 18 months in only three. However, by three years from surgery six cases of loosening had occurred with severe pain in the majority. The remaining joints loosened between three and five years from operation. The severity of the pain was irrespective of which component was loose. Typical symptoms appeared before x-ray changes were present, and the pain could be reproduced and accurately localized by the patient by gentle lateral stressing at examination. Usually this appraisal was sufficient to identify which component was loose before the full-blown radiological picture appeared. The loosening inevitably occurs at the cement bone interphase.

10. Revision for loosening. At revision surgery the loose component is usually removed with ease together with its cement sheath. If one of the components was tight it was nevertheless removed also (except in one case where a humeral component was left as a makeshift hemiarthoplasty articulating with the olecranon where it proved surprisingly stable). In this case it was decided that to remove the component would have severely damaged the humerus and the clinical result was satisfactory following this unusual salvage procedure. Two revised cases had another similar hinge inserted. Both cases loosened again within one year and the hinge was removed. One case subsequently had percutaneous Kirschner wire fixation, but stability was lost at three weeks and after removal of the wires the patient was left with a flail arm. The other patient achieved a better result with 90° of strong painfree motion and

good stability after the elbow had been fixed for six weeks maintaining bony apposition by use of transverse bone pins and an external clamp.

11. Five patients were revised by insertion of a new type of semi-constrained joint designed for these problems. (For description of joint see below.) The first two cases dislocated and this disaster led to modification in the design eliminating this complication. The clinical results in the three successful revisions (and in six other unreported cases where this joint has been inserted as a primary procedure) are encouraging at up to 18 months of surgery with an excellent range of motion and nothing to suggest further loosening despite the very poor bone found at surgery (Fig. 2).

The New Prosthesis (Fig. 3)

12. This newly designed semi-constrained joint used for revising the loose elbow hinge has a snap fit mechanism so essential when reconstructing a flail elbow. It gives immediate stability whilst any supporting soft tissue reconstruction is healing. However, when articulated it is polycentric and this allows for some error in placing the axis of rotation. Also, being a metal/high density polyethylene bearing, metal sensitivity problems are avoided. Finally, it allows for 15° of lateral deviation and some rotation (even in full extension), and it also has a built-in carrying angle of some 12° equally distributed between the humeral and ulna stems which make equal angles of inclination to the mean axis of rotation of the joint. (Subsequently, the joint has been further modified so that the previously flat metal plate forming a base supporting the ulnar plastic and bearing has now been curved to a convexity which lies more snugly within the contours of the sigmoid notch.)

DISCUSSION

13. The anxieties expressed by Souter (1973) are shown to be well founded. These results show this type of elbow hinge does not give durable good results beyond two years. The complications of the inplant are serious and salvage is difficult.

14. Much has been learned about joint replacement since the original prosthesis was designed (Ref.3). Metal bearings are now generally unacceptable and it is not surprising that of eight patients tested for loosening three subsequently exhibited metal sensitivity to chrome or nickel. Even replacing the bearing by a metal/plastic one cannot prolong the life of this joint. The failure of fully constrained hinge joints in the knee is now fully documented and were such a device as my original elbow hinge to be presented as a new design today for implantation, its failure would be predictable for exactly the same reasons.

15. By contrast, the new semi-constrained joint has an appropriate bearing surface, it is not fully constrained, it is polycentric and has a built-in ability to take up some lateral and rotary torque even in extension. We may hope it will give much more durable results and it is presently proving useful in salvaging flail joints and these difficult cases where a loose elbow hinge is removed. It is particularly useful where immediate stability must be provided and we are

tempted to reach for the hinge joint that we know will not give durable results. The new joint is sufficiently small to be inserted between the humeral epicondyles without their resection, but can equally be used where there is absence of portions of the distal humerus or proximal ulna. Thus, either the ligaments of the elbow joints can be used to give stability to the arthoplasty or where necessary some soft tissue reconstructive operation can be used as an adjunct.

CONCLUSIONS

16.   The elbow hinge which I introduced in 1972 is now obsolete. The results at 5 years show an unacceptably high incidence of loosening.

17.   The incidence of loosening increases noticeably after two years from implantation of the hinge.

18.   Search continues for a satisfactory primary implant. It may be that the solution will require two different kinds of elbow joints for the two different clinical problems. Thus, a satisfactory surface liner would be required for the architecturally good joint. A semi-constrained joint has been used and is presented for consideration when the problem is a flail limb with absence of bone stock or ligaments. Initial results using this joint are encouraging.

REFERENCES

1.   DEE R. 'Total replacement arthroplasty of the elbow for rheumatoid arthritis'. J. Bone Jt. Surgery, 1972, 54B, p. 88.

2.   DEE R. 'Total replacement of the elbow joint'. Modern Trends in Orthopaedics, Ed. Apley A.G., 1972, Butterworth p.250-265

3.   SOUTER W.A. 'Arthroplasty of the elbow'. Orthopaedic Clinics of North America, 1973, 4, n°2, p. 395.

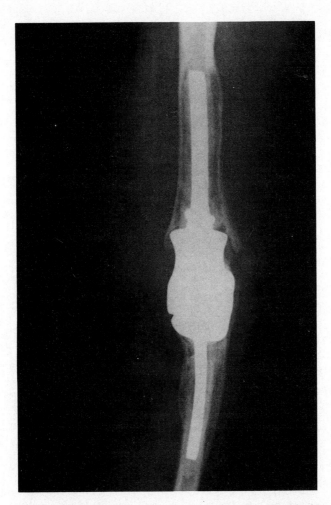

Fig. 1: A loose hinge 2½ years from surgery. Note the thinning of the cortex of the bone due to the abrading effect of loose cement

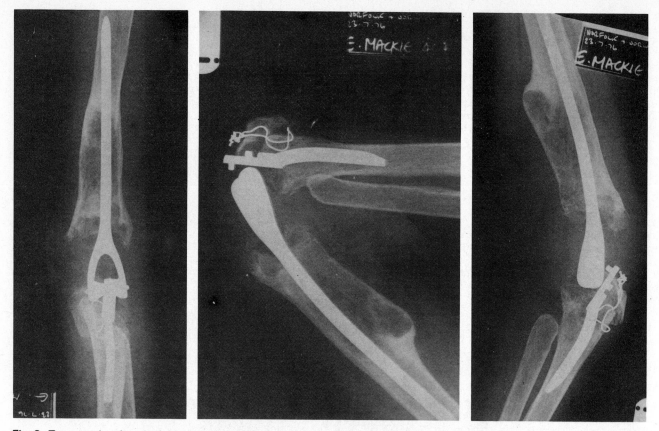

Fig. 2: Two months after the joint shown in Fig. 1 has been removed and replaced by the new semi-constrained joint. Note the excellent range of movement. The figures also show the gross damage to the bone caused by the previously loose hinge

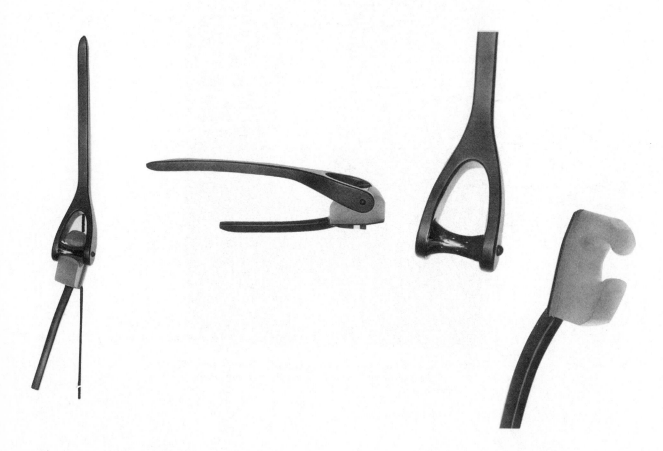

Fig. 3: The new semi constrained joint. For explanation see text

C163/77

A SIMPLE METHOD OF TOTAL ELBOW REPLACEMENT

M.E. CAVENDISH, MB, ChB, MChOrth, FRCS,
Whiston Hospital, Prescot, Lancashire

M.A. ELLOY, PhD, CEng, MIMechE,
Bio-Engineering and Medical Physics Unit, University of Liverpool, Liverpool

SYNOPSIS A simple, rationalised and relatively inexpensive humero-ulnar joint replacement has been designed, which gives adequate function and complete relief of pain to sufferers of osteo or rheumatoid arthritis of the elbow. The prosthesis which consists of a stainless steel trochlear replacement and an ultra-high-molecular-weight-polyethylene ulnar lining is cemented in place by means of a simple low trauma operation requiring minimum bone removal and giving maximum salvage potential. Natural ligaments are retained for stability. Although not essential for satisfactory insertion, special instruments have been designed which facilitate surgical accuracy.

1. INTRODUCTION

Severe arthritic changes are less common in the elbow than in the joint of the hand and of the lower limb. However, loss of elbow function can be more incapacitating, greatly impeding essential everyday actions such as eating and washing, and the use of crutches etc. The normal elbow consists of two distinct joints, one of these is the humero-ulnar joint between the trochlea of the humerus and the trochlear notch of the ulna, and the other is the humero-radial joint between the capitulum of the humerus and the head of the radius. The former, which is generally described as 'the true elbow joint' provides the function of the elbow flexion. The latter serves to carry compressive axial loads in the forearm, while providing for rotation (supination and pronation) of the hand. Clinical experience has shown that patients manage well, after a pseudarthrosis of the humero-radial joint by excision of the radial head. In these cases the load bearing function of this joint is taken over by the humero-ulnar joint and the interosseous membrane, which binds the ulna and the radius together. This fact is well recognised and has been frequently exploited in the design of elbow joint prostheses. The purpose of this paper is to describe a humero-ulnar prosthesis and the rationale behind its design.

2. DESCRIPTION OF PROSTHESIS

The prosthesis consists of two small parts, a humeral component made of stainless steel and an ulnar component made of ultra-high-molecular-weight-polyethylene, giving the essential feature of a low friction arthroplasty. Fig. 1. shows the humeral component which is 25 mm long, consists of a bobbin shape having 360° surface of revolution formed as two frustro-cones joined at their smaller ends, the major and minor diameters being 18.5 mm and 9.5 mm respectively. The end faces of the bobbin are mutually inclined at 20° and are provided with ribs 6 mm high and 1.5 mm thick diametrically placed in the plane of convergence. 6 mm wide notches are formed in these ribs along the axis of revolution. Fig. 2 shows the ulnar component, which is formed of a 160° sector of a 15 mm wide and 25 mm dia. cylinder, has coaxial internal bearing surfaces complementary to that of the trochlear component. Two 2 mm wide by 1.5 mm deep cement keying grooves are symmetrically formed in the outer surface parallel to the axis of revolution and a third, 6 mm wide tangential groove with a maximum depth of 4 mm is provided for additional cement keying and for the passage of a bone screw described later. The end faces of the ulnar component are chamfered as shown in Fig. 2. Placed together the two prosthetic components have a possible articulation range of 200°. Three jigging holes are provided in the plane faces of the ulnar component to accommodate the ulnar component holder described later and an X-ray marker fitted to the outer surface also aids fixation.

3. BASIC OPERATIVE PROCEDURE (Ref. Fig. 3)

3.1 Using no special instruments

The prosthesis was designed for insertion using the following simple operative procedure, requiring no special instruments.

A longitudinal incision is made posteriorly to expose the proximal end of the ulna and the ulnar nerve is mobilised and retracted to one side. The head of the radius is excised and a hole drilled axially through the olecranon into the medullary canal of the ulna. The olecranon is then divided transversely and folded back on the triceps tendon giving access to both the trochlea and the articular surfaces of the trochlear notch. The trochlea is excised by two saw cuts mutually inclined at 20° and passing into the olecranon and coracoid fossae, the width of this slot being sufficient to accommodate the prosthesis and about 1 mm of cement. The angle of the slot is also arranged to tilt the prosthesis axis of revolution in order to maintain the carrying angle.

Sufficient bone is removed from the area of the trochlear notch in both the ulna and olecranon to accommodate the plastic ulnar component and a trial reduction made using a trial prosthesis.

Some cancellous bone is gouged out of the

sides of the slot to provide a key for the cement. The humeral component is then cemented into position, the tapered ends of the prosthesis driving cement into the interstices of cancellous bone.

Cement is then pressed down the screw hole in the ulna, into the prepared cavity for the prosthesis and into the keying slots of the plastic component. The prosthesis is fitted and the olecranon fixed in position by a single 2½" bone screw through the drilled hole. The extension and flexion of the elbow are checked and pressure exerted on the olecranon to maintain reduction until the cement has hardened. The incision is then closed in layers without drainage. A tourniquet is used throughout.

4. SPECIAL INSTRUMENTATION

Although a satisfactory implantation may be made without the aid of special instruments, small components made slippery by contact with body fluids can be difficult to handle and accurately align. The special instruments shown in Fig. 4 were designed to overcome this difficulty.

4.1 Trochlear saw guide

This was designed to facilitate cutting of the prosthetic bed in the humerus. A peg on the hidden side of the blade locates in the notch of the natural trochlea. The handle is then aligned at the appropriate carrying angle to the extended axis of the ulna and an oscilating saw is used to cut along either side of the tapered blade of the saw guide, terminating in the olecranon and coracoid fossae. When the bone fragment is removed, the slot this produces accommodates the prosthesis and about 1 mm of cement when inserted to the correct depth.

4.2 Humeral component holder

To facilitate handling of this component the forceps shown were designed. These have PTFE jaws with a form complementary to the bearing surface of the prosthesis. These are used to position the prosthesis in its cement bed and protect the highly polished bearing suface during removal of excess cement. A separate plastic headed pusher is used to press the humeral prosthetic component firmly in position while the cement is hardening, without the risk of rocking (and thereby loosening) the prosthetic fixation.

4.3 Ulnar component holder

The plastic ulnar prosthesis has no pronounced linear feature such as a stem to clearly indicate its alignment in the ulna. Although satisfactory positioning can be achieved by eye, as in the first fifteen implantations, it was thought that a holding tool giving external indication of alignment could simplify the procedure. This tool, shown top left in Fig. 4 has two arms, one fixed and the other hinged, each provided with small pins which locate in the jigging holes of the ulnar prosthesis previously described. A latch holds the hinged arm in engagement with the prosthesis and a screw with a ball jointed slipper and tee handle can be made to advance perpendicularly towards the cementing surface of the prosthesis. A guide rod set mutually perpendicular to the screw and the axis of revolution of

the prosthesis, lies parallel to the ulna (or at a suitable carrying angle) when the prosthesis is correctly located in the bone. This instrument is used in the following manner.

After preparation of the cement bed in the ulna and olecranon, the prosthesis is mounted on the two jigging pins of the fixed arm of the holder. Cement is pressed with the bony bed and the keying grooves of the prosthesis. The prosthesis is hooked into position under the ulna and the hinged arm swung into engagement and latched in position. With the guide rod held parallel to the ulna, the prosthesis is pulled firmly into the cemented bed by means of the screw pressing against the outer cortex of the ulna. Excess cement is removed and the olecranon reattached by means of a single bone screw. After the cement has hardened, the instrument is removed by backing of the screw releasing the latched arm and disengaging the location pins of the fixed arm.

5. DESIGN CONSIDERATIONS

5.1 Articulation

The prosthesis was designed according to the philosophy described by Elloy et. al. (1) but specific considerations are described below. The natural elbow articulates as a simple hinge, whose axis tilts some 10 or 20 degrees during approximately 145° of active flexion. This conjunct rotation gives the so called 'carrying angle' of the straight arm shown in Fig. 3 while allowing alignment of upper and lower arm in full flexion. As pointed out by Kapandji (2) some elbows do not exhibit this conjunct rotation and others have greater rotation. However, the same effect can be produced by rotation of the humerus. The authors therefore considered that to preserve this characteristic would be an unjustified complication which would necessitate different prostheses for left and right elbows. They did however feel that the carrying angle should be maintained which precluded the use of an intra-medullary stem for its fixation if handedness was to be avoided.

In the normal joint, range of movement is usually controlled by the soft tissues and not by bony impingement. The authors considered that range of movement of the prosthesis should be sufficient to allow normal soft tissue limits to operate, otherwise incalculable stresses could be induced in the prosthesis and its fixation at the limits of articulation. By replacing the normal articular surfaces of the joint by similarly shaped prosthetic materials, a normal range of articulation with natural constraints has been maintained.

The articulating surfaces of the natural elbow are provided by the bobbin shaped trochlea and the complimentary shaped trochlear notch which encompasses about 180° of the trochlea. As shown in Fig. 5 the trochlea approximates to two frustrocones joined at their small ends and with their large ends blending into the epicondyles. This shape gives lateral stability, a characteristic which must be provided by the prosthetic replacement. The axis of the trochlea lies forward of the axis of the humeral shaft and approximately at right angles to it. Above the trochlea the coronoid and olecranon fossae, which are depressions in the front and back of the humerus leave only a thin web of bone supporting the central necked position of the trochlea and in many bones these fossae interconnect leaving the trochlea unsupported at its centre. Thus almost 360° of the surface of the trochlea is available for articulation. A twist on the trochlear form provides the conjunct rotation. By replacing the natural asymmetric trochlea by similarly proportioned prosthesis with a symmetrical shape, and having its axis of revolution suitably inclined, an articulation close to the natural elbow has been reproduced with natural lateral stability and maintenance of the 'carrying angle'. The symmetry achieved by eliminating the unnecessary conjunct rotation and the absence of an intramedullary stem allows the same prosthesis to be used in either arm.

Disengagement of the trochlea and trochlear notch is in nature resisted by the collateral ligaments which bridge the joint medially and laterally and are inserted into the epicondyles of the humerus close to the axis of articulation. Thus they stabilise the joint without restricting articulation and, because of their limited elasticity allow subluxation (partial dislocation) under abnormal or twisting load conditions. This feature serves to limit the mechanical forces that can be transmitted through the natural joint and also help to cushion the effects of suddenly applied loads. By retaining these natural stabilising features for the prosthesis, natural loading limits have been maintained.

5.2 Loading

Loads occurring in the elbow during normal activity are at present unknown and are difficult to ascertain accurately. However, there is considerable evidence in the literature to support the hyposthesis that living bone remodels to accommodate imposed loads. It is also reasonable to assume that, even in the diseased joint, the adjacent bony structures are capable of supporting and distributing natural loading. Referring to Fig. 5, joint loads are normally transmitted from the trochlea to the humeral shaft by the trabeculae of the epicondyles and of the supracondylar ridges. In addition to distributing the forces, these cancellous bone structures, by virtue of their viscoelastic properties, have a capacity to absorb energy in shock loading.

By ensuring near natural load levels on the prosthesis and by using the natural load distributing structures we can expect bone stresses to be tolerable, provided that efficient fixation is achieved. The tapered ends of the prosthetic trochlea are designed to drive acrylic bone cement, which is used for its fixation, into the interstices of the cancellous bone of the epicondyles Fig. 3, 5 and 6. It is hoped that by this method, firm fixation with optimum load distribution has been attained. Of course, cement is not an adhesive, but merely a filling agent so that ribs and notches on the prosthesis are necessary for keying purposes and the distribution of anterio-posterior loads on the humeral component.

On the ulnar side the articular surfaces of the trochlear notch are somewhat complimentary to those of the trochlea and load is naturally transmitted to the shaft through a thin cortex and underlying cancellous bone. By removing only sufficient bone to accommodate the prosthesis and a small quantity of acrylic cement, as shown

in Figure 3, and then firmly keying the cement to the remaining cancellous bone it is expected that firm fixation may be achieved together with optimum load distribution.

5.3 Salvageability

A satisfactory salvage procedure must be available in case of failure, be this due to infection or technical reasons. If infection occurred the only course of action would be the removal of the implant and the creation of a pseudarthrosis (false joint). For a material failure, removal of all or part of the implant and replacement by a suitable alternative may be the optimum salvage procedure. This design has been aimed to allow shallow fixation with minimal bone removal and retention of the ligaments, in order to give the maximum scope for satisfactory salvage. Other total elbow prostheses described in the literature, such as that in Fig. 6, entail substantial bone removal and elimination of stabilising ligaments during their insertion. They also employ long intramedullary stems for their fixation making satisfactory salvage much more difficult to achieve.

5.4 Surgery

Another design objective was to permit a simple operative procedure without the need for special purpose instrumentation. This has been achieved, the first fifteen prostheses having been satisfactorily implanted without the aid of such instruments. However, it was considered that the surgery could be facilitated and accuracy enhanced by the provision of a limited number of special instruments, which were designed and used in later operations. Although the prosthesis was designed for a specific operative approach, it was recognised that orthopaedic surgeons express a great measure of individuality in their techniques and that the prescribed approach may not be best suited in all cases. Flexibility of surgical techniques was therefore a significant design consideration.

6. MECHANICAL TESTS

The authors had some difficulty in deciding what meaningful in vitro testing of the prosthesis could be conducted and a shortage of suitable biological material placed severe constraints on them.

6.1 Friction and wear

Such tests are expensive to set up, take a long time to complete and are of questionable validity in the absence of quantitative load data for the elbow joint. This prosthesis design concept provides a bearing surface configuration and area comparable with that of the natural joint, and for reasons already explained loading is also expected to be similar to that occurring in the natural joint. Charnley type total hip replacement, employing the same material combination as this prosthesis but having bearing surface areas approximately one quarter to that of the natural joint, have been subjected to exhaustive in vitro wear testing at several centres. These tests and subsequent clinical experience have shown that prostheses of this type have adequate wear life. Wear-out of this new elbow prosthesis is not therefore expected to be a problem and so wear tests were not undertaken.

6.2 Strength

Because of the shallow fixation adopted, the strength of the prosthetic components themselves was expected to be far greater than that of the bone – cement, or cement – prosthesis interfaces. Each of the prosthetic components can only be loaded by the other and because of its limited bearing surface, the ulnar component may only be substantially loaded in a direction that presses it into its cemented bed, although a limited lateral force may be also applied. The humeral component on the other hand may be loaded in a number of directions and is therefore more vunerable to dislodgement. However, because prosthetic stability is imparted by natural ligaments, forces must be limited to those which will cause dislocation of the joint.

The fixation of the humeral component might be expected to be weakest when loaded downwards along the humeral shaft, i.e. opposite to its direction of insertion. Active loading in this direction is however limited to the lifting ability of the subject. One might expect the most vunerable loading direction of the humeral component to be backward, i.e. perpendicular to the humeral shaft, such a load may only be applied by axial loading along the ulna with the elbow flexed to 90° a condition which might occur if the subject were checking a fall. In this case the force could be limited only by dislocation of the joint. With only three fresh cadaveric elbows at their disposal, the authors decided to use these in an attempt to measure
a) the force to cause posterior dislocation of the natural elbow at 90° of flexion after the radial head had been excised.
b) the force to dislodge the humeral component applied downwards along the humeral axis.
c) the backward force perpendicular to the humeral shaft, which will dislodge the humeral component.
The test specimens had approximately 2 – 3 inches of humeral and ulnar shafts attached, which were cast into blocks of plastic for mounting in the test machine. A Howden 10 kN universal testing machine was used for this purpose. All the ligaments were kept intact although no attempt was made to simulate muscle forces. Disarticulated humeral prosthetic loads were applied through the medium of a separate ulnar prosthetic component.

The force to dislocate the natural elbow measured on the first specimen was 1.26 kN at which point the coronoid process fractured. An attempt to repeat this test on the second specimen resulted in fracture of the humeral shaft at 1.2 kN. On the first specimen the force to pull out the humeral component in the direction of the humeral axis was 0.7 kN, failure being at the cement – bone interface. Posterior dislodgement was achieved on the third specimen at 1.5 kN, when transverse splitting of the epicondyles occurred in the plane of symmetry of the prosthesis.

7. CLINICAL RESULTS

At the time of writing twenty prostheses had been implanted, fifteen of these were implanted with-

out the use of special instruments and the remainder using the instruments described. Two had to be removed but the others have remained satisfactory. Ten of these cases have a 1½ – 3 year follow up and include the two failures. One of which was removed because of post-operative infection and the other because of fracture of the humerus resulting from the use of crutches. Both of these were successfully salvaged by pseudarthrosis producing a painless joint with a good range of movement. The other eight cases have adequate range of movement the best giving 5 – 135° of flexion and the worst giving 40° – 110° of flexion. All are pain free even though some patients are using walking aids such as crutches, sticks etc.

8. FURTHER DEVELOPMENT

Ways of enhancing fixation in severely eroded bone are currently under consideration. These, shown in Fig. 7, include extension of the keying ribs of the humeral component both laterally into the epicondyle and proximally into the supracondylar ridges. This could help to prevent spreading of the supracondylar ridges during axially applied forces. An alternative suggestion, to achieve fixation by enclosing the condyles, was rejected on two counts. Firstly, this would make the prosthesis subcutaneous with its inherent problems of wound healing and skin breakdown and secondly clinical experience with the Smith Peterson Cup prosthesis suggests that necrosis of cancellous bone enclosed in cement would occur. A small anterior projection on the plastic ulnar component shown in Fig. 7 was also considered for improved keying into the cement. However this has not been adopted as no post operative loosening of the component has yet occurred.

9. CONCLUSION

A simple, rationalised and relatively inexpensive prosthetic design has been achieved capable of restoring adequate pain-free function to severely disabled osteo or rheumatoid arthritic elbows, employing a simple low trauma operation and giving the maximum salvage potential in the event of failure. Although satisfactory implantation may be achieved without the aid of special purpose instruments, four such instruments have been designed to simplify the procedure and facilitate accuracy of insertion.

REFERENCES

1. Elloy M.A., Wright J.T.M., and Cavendish M.E., The basic requirements and design criteria for total joint prostheses. Acta orthop. scand. 47, 193-202, 1976.

2. Kapandji I.A. The physiology of the joints. V.I. 1st edition 1970 (Longman Group, London)

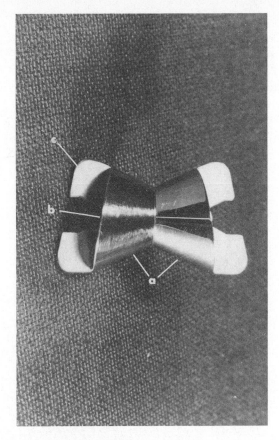

Fig. 1: Liverpool Prosthesis — humeral component
  a) conical articular surfaces
  b) mutually inclined cementation faces
  c) cementation ribs

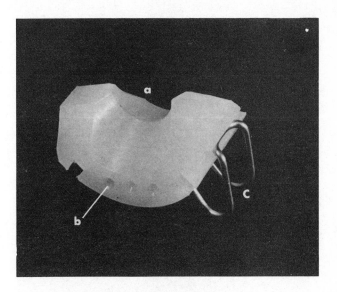

Fig. 2: Liverpool Elbow — ulnar component
  a) UHMWP component
  b) instrumentation jigging holes
  c) metal X-ray marker

Fig. 3: Liverpool Prosthesis — implanted position
  A) carrying angle
  a) ulnar, b) humerus, c) radial head excised,
  d) coronoid and olecranon fossae, e) cement,
  f) ulnar axis, g) humeral axis

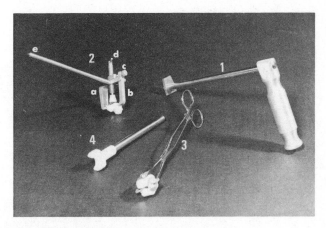

Fig. 4: Prototype instrumentation for Liverpool Elbow
  (1) Trochlear saw guide
  (2) Ulnar component holder — with ulnar prosthesis
      a) fixed arm
      b) hinged arm
      c) latch
      d) clamping screw
      e) guide rod
  (3) Humeral component holder—with humeral prosthesis
  (4) Pusher

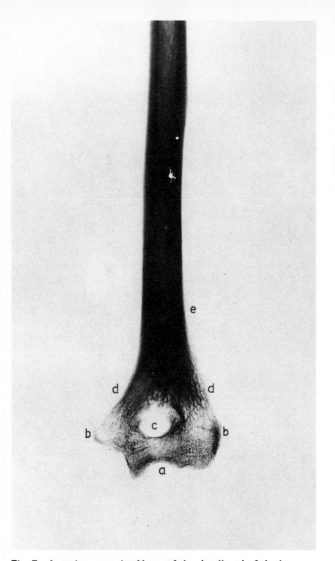

Fig. 5: Anterior-posterior X-ray of the detail end of the humerus
showing   a) trochlea
          b) epicondyles
          c) coronoid and olecranon fossae
          d) supracondylar ridges
          e) humeral shaft

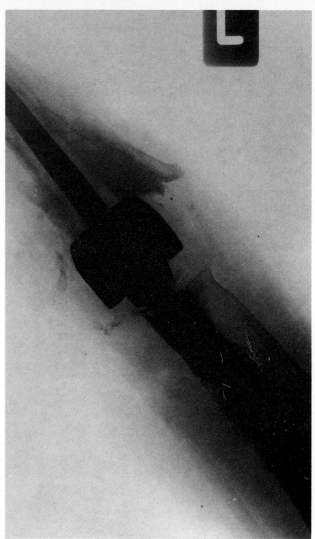

Fig. 6: Anterior-posterior X-ray of a prosthetic elbow showing
the typical long intramedullary stems

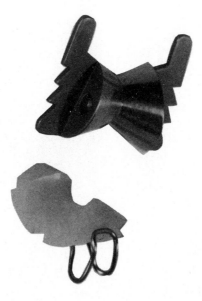

Fig. 7: Modified Liverpool Elbow Prosthesis showing extended
cementation ribs on ulnar component and cementation
stem on ulnar component

TOTAL REPLACEMENT ARTHROPLASTY OF THE ELBOW

W.A. SOUTER, MB, ChB, FRCSEd
Arthritis Unit, Princess Margaret Rose Orthopaedic Hospital,
and Royal Infirmary, Edinburgh

INTRODUCTION

1. When the orthopaedic history of our era comes to be written, the 1960's will almost certainly be remembered as the decade in which the endeavours to produce a successful and durable hip arthroplasty were finally brought to fruition. Following in the wake of this success, the 1970's are witnessing an enormous upsurge of interest in the replacement of other joints, including the elbow.

2. At the turn of the decade, several hinge prostheses for the elbow became available in this country, and between 1969 and 1972, 30 of these operations were performed in the Arthritis Unit in Edinburgh. It is the purpose of this paper to review the results achieved in these cases with particular reference to the main complications and problems which have arisen and to report on a research project aimed at designing a different type of prosthesis which hopefully might be less prone to the problems which have beset hinge arthroplasty.

REVIEW SERIES DATA

3. The review series comprises 22 patients, 5 of whom had bilateral surgery, from the author's own unit and 2 patients from that of the late Douglas Savill, one of these being bilateral. 21 of the patients were suffering from rheumatoid arthritis, one from osteoarthritis and three had had failed fascial arthroplasties. As might be expected in a series of predominantly rheumatoid cases, two thirds of the patients were female. The ages ranged from 33 to 71 years (mean 57 years).

4. By far the most common clinical indication for surgery was severe intractable pain, this being present in 28 of the elbows operated on. Other major complaints were instability (12 cases), major loss of movement (10 cases) and marked persistent synovial swelling (15 cases). All the elbows showed severe grade 4 or 5 erosions on radiological examination (Ref. 5).

5. The implants used in the series were the original McKee hinge in 23, the modified McKee with its shorter, recontoured stems in 1, the Dee in 5, and the Shiers in 1 (Ref. 3 and 1). The operative technique was as described by McKee and Souter (Ref. 3 and 6).

RESULTS

6. Two of the patients in the original series have died from unrelated causes, one of these patients having bilateral implants. Two other patients have required to have their prostheses removed because of secondary infection and in the final analysis will be added to the poor results of the series (Para. 18 and Table 5). There remain 25 elbows on which a four to six year follow-up (mean 5 yrs. 3 months) is now available and an important feature of the review is the comparison of the results pertaining at one year after operation with those at the time of the final review.

PATIENTS' OWN ASSESSMENT

7. If we look first of all at the subjective results following hinge arthroplasty, we find that at the time of the final review, 18 of the 25 elbows are still considered by the patients themselves to have been markedly improved with regard to pain status. At the other end of the scale, however, there are 5 patients who have already required revision because of the severity of the persisting discomfort.

8. With regard to elbow function, the subjective assessment is rather less impressive, only 12 of the elbows being considered as markedly improved and some 8 cases as either worse or already requiring revision.

OBJECTIVE ASSESSMENT OF RESULTS

Pain Status

9. Whereas 23 of the elbows pre-operatively were the seat of severe pain, 16 were rendered completely free of pain in the immediate post-operative period, and even at the final review this figure is being fairly well maintained, 14 having no pain and 3 only occasional pain (Table 1). There is, however, a definite element of deterioration in that whereas at 1 year only 3 patients had severe pain, 6 now come into this category.

Range of Movement

10. With regard to the range of movement, pre-operatively all save 2 patients had less than 110° of movement, 6 having less than 50°. Post-operatively however, 15 patients achieved more than 110° of movement and only 1 patient had less than 90° (Table 2). Again however there has been a slight element of deterioration in that at the final review, only 10

patients now have more than 110° of movement and 5 patients have less than 90°. This tendency is also confirmed by the mean range of movement calculated for the series as a whole at the three observation intervals; pre-operatively 73°, 1 year after operation 114°, and final review 103°.

MAIN LONG TERM PROBLEMS

11. In spite of this tendency towards gradual deterioration, it might be thought that, in view of the reasonably satisfactory maintenance of pain relief and an acceptable range of motion in a very sizeable proportion of the patients, hinge arthroplasty could be recommended with a fair degree of confidence in rheumatoid patients with severely destroyed elbows. This, however, is very far from the truth, since careful follow-up over the years has shown that this procedure is by no means devoid of significant complications (Ref. 6, 7, 8). In particular, it can give rise to three serious long-term problems viz. a) loosening of the implant, especially in the humerus, leading to clinical instability, b) danger of fracture as a result of resorption of bone in the lower humerus and c) gross instability in the event of the prosthesis having to be removed.

a) Loosening of the prosthesis

12. The radiological evidence for loosening of the implants has been graded in 5 categories (Table 3). The thin linear translucency around the cement plug characteristic of Grade 2 may be of doubtful significance but there is no question that the wide translucency of Grade 3 signifies a loose joint. Grade 4 is characterised by some degree of cortical erosion and penetration of the loose hinge into the medullary cavity of the humerus, while in Grade 5 there is marked thinning of the humeral cortex, impending perforation, and ballooning of the contour of the bone (Fig. 1). At one year after operation, 13 of the 25 elbows showed either no evidence of loosening or only a linear translucency around the cement plug, whereas at the final review only 4 came into this category. At the other extreme, whereas only 2 cases showed marked loosening at one year, no less than 12 are in this situation now.

13. The severer grades of radiological loosening are associated with a greater or lesser degree of clinical instability. This latter problem has also been classified into 5 grades - none, just detectable on passive movement, unstable but well controlled on active movement, marked instability with only limited function and finally gross clinical instability. The incidence of these grades is shown in Table 4. Whereas at 1 year post operation, 16 patients were essentially stable, only 5 come into these favourable categories at the final review. At the other end of the scale, whereas only 4 patients were unstable at 1 year after operation, no less than 11 exhibit major instability at the present time.

Causes for high incidence of loosening

14. The author would submit that a number of factors may contribute to the high incidence of loosening.

(i) Normally with cement fixation of implants in the lower limb, the cement plug is impacted against the bone under normal conditions of loading. In the distal humerus, however, especially during lifting, it is clear that distracting forces may operate between the cement plug and the endosteal bone.

(ii) Certain activities exemplified by the holding of a moderately heavy weight between the opposed palms of the hands with the elbows flexed to 90° are liable to transmit major rotational forces from the forearm to the humerus. Normally these are absorbed and transmitted by the trochlear and radio-capitellar joints supported by the important 'tie-beam' of the medial collateral ligament which prevents opening of the medial side of the elbow. Once the epicondyles have been removed however, and with them the collateral ligaments, rotational forces transmitted via a fully constrained hinge must perforce be concentrated at the cement/bone interface in the humerus.

(iii) Supination and pronation may also generate rotational forces which may have some effect on the humeral fixation but are more likely to be concentrated at the cement/bone interface in the ulna. It is indeed of interest that with a longer follow-up, loosening in the ulna is now becoming apparent in an increasing number of patients.

(iv) The pull of the common flexor muscles and of the brachioradialis with the elbow at 90° must inevitably tend to displace the forearm backwards relative to the longitudinal axis of the humerus and as a result, angle the tip of the humeral stem forwards against the anterior cortex. That this may indeed play a role in loosening of the prosthesis is suggested by at least 2 cases in the series where impending perforation of the anterior humeral cortex by the tip of the stem of a Dee prosthesis has been observed on X ray.

(v) Two patients in the series with striking evidence of loosening have been shown on patch testing to be sensitive to cobalt. Thus, in a few cases, non-mechanical factors may contribute to loosening of the implant.

(b) Danger of fracture

15. Where the lower end of the humerus has become thin and ballooned as in Fig. 1, a fall on the point of the elbow is likely to result in a comminuted fracture. Even with lesser degrees of bone erosion and resorption, a fracture may result from quite minor trauma (Fig. 2). Four fractures have occured so far in the series, two of them being severely comminuted. The first of these comminuted lesions healed on conservative treatment in plaster and a body bandage within 12 weeks, but in the second case, the result was less satisfactory. Conservative treatment failed to produce healing and even after open reduction, internal fixation, re-cementing, and bone grafting, only a painless pseudarthrosis was obtained.

(c) Gross instability on removal of prosthesis

16. The original operative procedure necessitated by the type of hinges used in this series involves the removal of the epicondyles. Thus, in the event of the prosthesis having to be removed, as has happened in 2 patients because of secondary infection, there is no wide lower end of humerus to form a stable

articulation with the trochlear notch of the ulna and gross instability with a virtually flail elbow is likely to result (Fig. 3). In one of these patients no less than 180° of rotational instability were present at the elbow. Such a situation is extremely difficult to control satisfactorily with a splint. Indeed, in both of the cases in this series, stabilisation with any hinged splint was found to be impossible, and a carefully moulded polythene cast to maintain the elbow at 90° was all that could be offered.

OVERALL ASSESSMENT OF RESULTS

17. In view of the complications described above, it is clear that any assessment of elbow arthroplasty if it is to be really meaningful, must take account of pain status, function and stability. In the present review, five parameters have been used viz. pain status, extension loss, maximum flexion, total range of movement and clinical instability. On the basis of these criteria, the overall results have been classified as excellent, very good, good, fair and poor. The details of this assessment grading are listed by Souter (Ref. 8).

18. Whereas pre-operatively all the elbows were classified as poor, post-operatively no less than 18 came into the upper 3 gradings, all of which can be regarded as very acceptable clinical results (Table 5). At the final review, however, only 10 elbows are still in these categories, while 9 patients are now regarded as poor. Where an elbow in the fair or poor category exhibits painful instability, it may be necessary for the patient to wear a hinged polythene brace permanently.

CONCLUSIONS WITH REGARD TO HINGE ARTHROPLASTY

19. The tendency for gradual deterioration to occur after hinge arthroplasty and the potential of this operation to give rise to serious complications or even frank disasters render it unsuitable for routine use. It may however still have a very limited place where there is severe pain in a patient over the age of 65 with grade 4 or 5 X ray changes, where gross instability exists either primarily or following excision arthroplasty, or where there is bilateral ankylosis especially with shoulder involvement. Finally, it might occasionally be of use after severe elbow injury.

WHAT OF THE FUTURE?

20. In view of this rather disappointing conclusion, we must necessarily ask what alternative procedures are available for dealing with the severely destroyed elbow. A recent review of synovectomy and debridement of the elbow and of fascial arthroplasty by the author (Ref. 9) suggests that while these procedures have their place in properly selected cases, they provide no satisfactory substitute for a really good arthroplasty in the late rheumatoid patient. We are thus presented with the challenge of designing an elbow prosthesis which will not only ensure an excellent early result but will have the attribute of durability and 'salvagability'. In considering this problem, it is necessary to look again at the cumulative defects of the original type of hinge

implant. These are the loss of the humeral epicondyles and the collateral ligaments the marked tendency for loosening at the cement/bone interface, especially in the humerus, the severe endosteal erosion and resorption which may follow loosening of the prosthesis, the resultant danger of fracture the potential for extensive bone involvement on both sides of the joint should infection occur and the gross instability of the pseudarthrosis should the implant have to be removed.

POSSIBLE SOLUTIONS

21. Three approaches to these problems would seem to be worth considering.

(a) The use of a very slim hinge inserted between the epicondyles, thus leaving the collateral ligaments intact (Ref. 2, 4). It would seem to the author that while this may alleviate the problem of loosening, it is unlikely to abolish it.

(b) The use of a partially constrained hinge which would reduce the rotational stresses transmitted to the cement/bone interface. While this might well solve some of the problems, it still implies the use of stemmed implants with their unfortunate potential for extensive bone involvement either by erosion or infection if progress goes awry.

(c) The design of a partially constrained two-component metal on plastic joint fixed locally in the condyles of the humerus and ulna so that bone resection is minimal and ligamentous stability hopefully preserved

22. This last approach has over the past few years been the subject of a joint research project conducted in the Bioengineering Unit of the University of Strathclyde and the author's own arthritis service in Edinburgh.

DESIGN OF PROPOSED IMPLANT

23. In a preliminary morphological study of the elbow, it became apparent that the alignment and contour of the humeral/ulnar articulation were far from simple and the philosophy guiding our approach to the design of the new prosthesis has been not only to fashion the alignment and contours of the articular surfaces as closely as possible to the pattern of the normal trochlea, but also to determine the siting and dimensions of the fixation flanges by reference to the exact position of the surrounding bony buttresses. The proposed joint is based essentially on the bone model illustrated in Fig. 4, which itself was prepared by excising the surrounding bone from the trochlear articulation while leaving sufficient protruding medullary flanges as possible fixation devices

Articular surfaces

24. The resulting implant is a two-component metal on plastic prosthesis replacing only the trochlear articulation. It is envisaged that the head of the radius will in most cases be excised. The contour and alignment of the humeral component mimic very closely those of the normal trochlea, and like the latter are designed in such a way that on fixation of the implant the shoulders of the trochlea will be set at an oblique inclination to the sagittal plane. The articular surfaces of the humeral component are convex in the sagittal

plane but in the coronal reproduce the corresponding contour of the normal trochlea i.e. its medial surface is convex while its lateral surface is concave.

25. The ulnar component will be generally complementary to this and again will mimic the contours of the trochlear notch of the ulna (Fig. 4 and 5).

26. The closely matched saddle resulting from the above design should confer valuable inherent stability on the prosthesis and yet allow a certain amount of release 'glide' in both compartments when the ulna is subjected to any axial twisting action. We would also hope that by holding closely to the anatomical pattern, the normal role of the collateral ligaments would be preserved and thus any excess displacement resulting from rotational or angulating forces would be checked, as in the normal elbow, by the opposing medial or lateral ligament (Fig. 5).

Fixation of implant

27. The probable role of rotational forces in the loosening of hinge prostheses has already been stressed (paragraph 14). The retention of the medial and lateral ligaments in the proposed arthroplasty should help to reduce the transmission of these forces to the cement/bone interface, but as an adjunct to this, the fixation flanges have been designed in such a way that the humeral component is secured over as wide an area of the intercondylar bone as possible.

28. The normal trochlea is heavily buttressed on its lateral side by the large bulk of the capitellum and excavation of the latter provides an ideal cavity in which a fairly long and substantial metal flange can be cemented. The medial side of the trochlea is less well buttressed, as the medial epicondyle comes off well posteriorly and fairly high up on the medial trochlear lip. Nevertheless, by siting a slim elliptical flange at an appropriate level on the prosthesis, good fixation can also be achieved medially. It is to be noted that the normal anatomy precludes the medial and lateral flanges being in the same coronal plane. The lateral can indeed be essentially coronal in alignment but the medial flange must be angled back from this plane.

29. Initially, it had been felt that the above fixation might have been sufficient. Later, however, it was decided that, as a safeguard against rotational forces about the coronal axis, a metal arch should be incorporated to secure the device to the excavated supracondylar ridges. Again the normal anatomy has determined the design of this arch. The supracondylar arch does not itself lie in the coronal plane but is positioned posteriorly relatively to the coronal axis of the trochlea on its medial side so as to become confluent with the medial epicondyle. Moreover, its lateral limb ascends almost vertically from the capitellum while its medial limb lies much more obliquely as it comes round the margin of the olecranon fossa (Fig. 4). Thus a symmetrically fashioned Y-fixation device would not measure up to the stringent anatomical criteria on which the present design concept has been built up. It is envisaged that three sizes may be necessary so as to ensure that the dimension of the arch matches any given supracondylar ridge sufficiently accurately to allow the metal to be counter sunk in the bone and thus avoid

the excessive bone cement loading which would result if it were too superficial.

30. These design criteria coupled to the 'saddle' contour of the articular surfaces will also mean that right and left sided implants will be necessary.

31. It had been hoped that the ulnar component might be secured by a single dovetailed posterior flange cemented axially in the olecranon Experience with rheumatoid elbows has shown, however that the olecranon is frequently so eroded as to consist only of the posterior cortex of the original bone. Thus, it has been necessary to supplement the original idea with a short ulnar stem inclined to the radial side of the longitudinal axis of the main articular surface to match the lie of the medullary cavity of the proximal ulna. The necessary length of this stem has been assessed by mechanical testing

32. The local fixation outlined above has been tested in cadaver studies to the point of failure and it appears that it should be sufficient to withstand the normal stresses operating across the elbow joint. These have been measured in the course of collateral studies on the biomechanics of the elbow carried out by Mr. A.C. Nicol of Strathclyde University.

SUMMARY

(a) Hinge arthroplasty of the elbow although capable of yielding highly successful results initially, lacks durability and in the event of total failure, 'salvagability'.

(b) The main problems arising from the procedure are loosening of the implant, danger of severe comminuted fracture in the thinned lower humerus and gross instability in the event of the prosthesis having to be removed.

(c) As a result of these problems, the indications for hinge arthroplasty of the McKee, Dee or Shiers type must be regarded as very limited.

(d) A new design concept for a locally fixed, partially constrained, two-component metal on plastic joint is described. This implant has been designed to mimic the normal anatomy of the articular surface of the human elbow and in so doing to preserve, as far as possible, ligamentous action.

(e) The proposed fixation for this new device is part and parcel of the uniform anatomical concept in that the siting and dimensions of the fixation flanges are accurately matched to the various bony buttresses which surround the trochlear articulation.

ACKNOWLEDGEMENTS

The author would like to stress that the development of the implant described above has been carried out in conjunction with Professor John P. Paul, Dr. N. Berme and Mr. A.C. Nicol of the Bioengineering Dept. of the University of Strathclyde. The bioengineering aspects of the project have been supported by a grant from the Arthritis and Rheumatism Council.

1.   DEE, R. Total replacement arthroplasty of the elbow for rheumatoid arthritis. J.Bone Jt. Surg. 54B: 88-95, 1972.

2.   GSCHWEND, N. Arthroplasty of the elbow using the GSB prosthesis.   Proceedings of the 12th Congress of the International Society of Orthopaedic Surgery & Traumatology, Tel-Aviv 1972. pp. 883-885. Excerpta Medica, Amsterdam 1973.

3.   McKEE, G.K. Total replacement of the elbow joint. Ibid. pp. 891-893. Excerpta Medica, Amsterdam 1973.

4.   MAZAS, F. et de la CAFFINIERE, J.-Y. Prosthèse totale de coude. Ibid. pp. 886-8. Excerpta Medica, Amsterdam 1973.

5.   PORTER, B.B., RICHARDSON, C. and VAINIO, K. Rheumatoid Arthritis of the Elbow: The results of synovectomy. J. Bone Jt. Surg. 56B: 427-437, 1974.

6. SOUTER, W.A. Arthroplasty of the Elbow. With particular reference to Metallic Hinge Arthroplasty in Rheumatoid patients. Orthop. Clin. N.America 4: 395-413, 1973.

7. SOUTER, W.A. Total metallic hinge arthroplasty of the rheumatoid elbow. Proceedings of the 12th Congress of the International Society of Orthopaedic Surgery and Traumatology. pp.889-890. Excerpta Medica, Amsterdam 1973.

8. SOUTER, W.A. Hinge Arthroplasty of the Elbow (in press).

9.   SOUTER, W.A. Conservative Surgery of the Rheumatoid Elbow (in press).

TABLE 1

PAIN STATUS

	Pre-op	1 year Post-op	Final Review *
No pain	1	16	14
Occasional pain		4	3
Mild, intermittent pain	1	2	2
Severe incapacitating pain	23	1	1
Revision required because of pain	–	2	5
	25	25	25

* 4-6 years 3 months. Mean 5 years 3 months (S.D. 7 months)

TABLE 2

ELBOW FUNCTION - RANGE OF MOVEMENT

	Pre-op	1 year Post-op	Final Review*
130° or more	2	5	2
110-129	–	10	8
90-109	8	9	10
50-89	9	1	5
50	6	–	–
	25	25	25

* 4-6 years 3 months. Mean 5 years 3 months (S.D. 7 months)

TABLE 3

X-RAY EVIDENCE OF LOOSENING

		1 year post-op	Final review *
Grade 1	Normal	5	4
2	Linear translucency	8	
3	Wide translucency	5	6
4	Cortical erosion	5	3
5	Marked thinning of cortex and/or impending perforation	2	12
		25	25

* 4-6 years 3 months. Mean 5 years 3 months (S.D. 7 months).

TABLE 4

DEGREE OF CLINICAL INSTABILITY

Grade	1 year post-op	Final review*
1	14	4
2	2	1
3	5	9
4	2	9
5	2	2
	25	25

* 4-6 years 3 months. Mean 5 years 3 months (S.D. 7 months)

TABLE 5

GENERAL ASSESSMENT OF RESULTS

Grade	1 year post-op	Final review *
Excellent	3	1
Very good	8	4
Good	7	5
Fair	4	8
Poor	5	9
	27	27

Note this table includes the 2 patients from whom the prostheses had to be removed because of secondary infection.

* 4-6 years 3 months. Mean 5 years 3 months (S.D. 7 months)

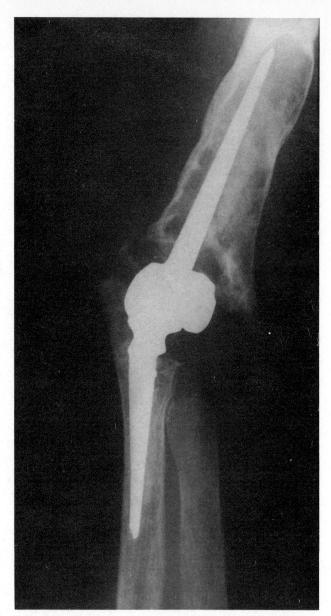

Fig. 1: Grade 5 loosening after hinge arthroplasty. Note the marked thinning and ballooning of the humeral cortex

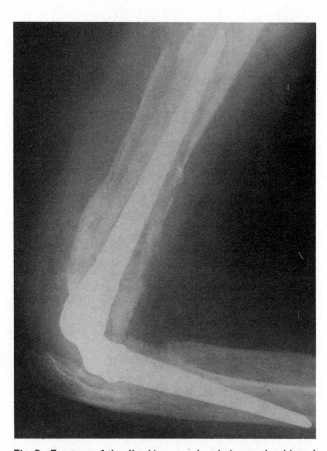

Fig. 2: Fracture of the distal humerus in relation to the thinned bone around the loose cement plug. This occurred as a result of a fall, five and a half years after insertion of the implant

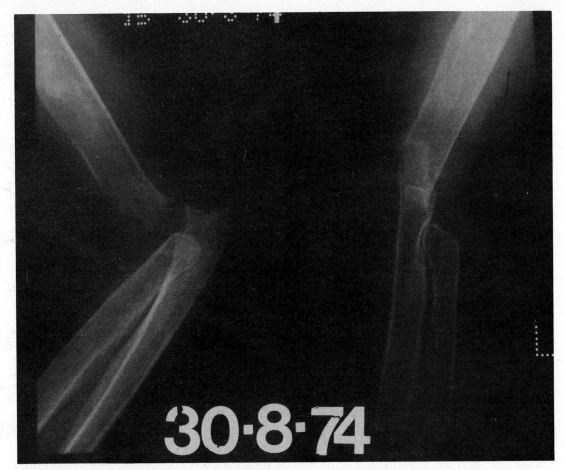

Fig. 3: Grossly unstable pseudarthrosis resulying from removal of Dee prosthesis. This patient had suffered secondary infection of the arthroplasty through a ruptured olecranon bursa

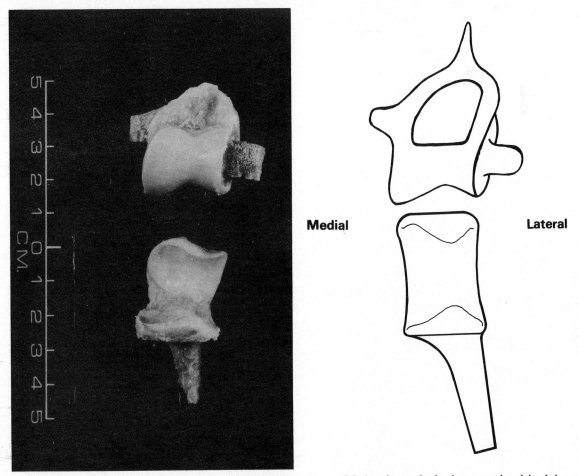

Medial   Lateral

Fig. 4: Bone model on which the design concept of the Strathclyde—Edinburgh prosthesis, shown on the right, is based

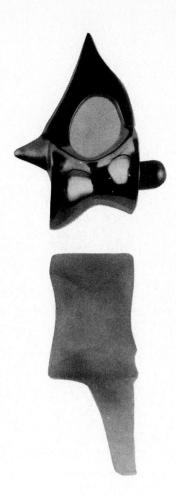

Fig. 5: Proposed design of new elbow prosthesis

GSB ELBOW-, WRIST-, AND PIP-JOINTS

N. GSCHWEND, H. SCHEIER, A. BÄHLER

GSB joints (GSB are the initials of the three designers Gschwend, Scheier and Bähler) are designed to allow the best possible physiological movement with good stability and a minimum of bone resection, so that in the event of complications retreat is possible by the conventional methods.

Initially a constrained hinge was used for the case of the elbow.Unfortunately, approximately one third of the 40 implanted GSB joints were subject to loosening a short time after the operation (one to five years). The causes will be discussed and a new GSB joint described.

With its design, the GSB wrist-joint simulates the really complex movement mechanism of the human wrist joint. As the analysis of the results shows, the design principle has proven successful. Nevertheless, because of difficulties in anchoring, an improved bearing surface must be provided..

The GSB Metacarpo-phalangeal-joint (MP-joint) is a prosthesis which can be fixed in the marrow cavity with the aid of a screw-like socket. To protect the anchoring arrangement, the metal pins of the prosthesis are allowed to move - like a piston - to and fro in the polyethylene sockets.

The GSB Proximal-interphalangeal-joint (PIP-joint) is a loosely connected hinged joint with a wide bearing surface and requires only slight intercondylar bone resection at the head of the proximal phalanx. A special enamel-metal coating of the marrow cavity pins is intended to make the use of cement superfluous. Results to date are reported.

GSB ELBOW-, WRIST-, MP- AND PIP-JOINTS

The design of our GSB joints has the following objectives:

1. To come as near as possible to the physiology of the joint to be replaced.

2. To provide both stability and mobility at the same time.

3. To resect as little bone as possible.

4. To retain the ligament and muscle insertions as far as possible, so that

5. In the event of complications, a wide path of retreat can be left open for other arthroplasties, expecially the simple resection arthroplasty or an arthrodesis.

The following remarks are intended to illustrate to what extent we have been able to meet these ambitious goals or to explain the reasons for failure.
One by one, the paper considers the design principle, operation technique, results, failures and their probable causes in respect of the GSB-elbow and wrist joint, and finally provides a brief introduction to our MP- and PIP-joints.

The GSB elbow-joint

A careful analysis of our 27 resection arthroplasties showed satisfactory results for the majority of cases after an average of six years after the operation. However, nine patients, i.e. one third of those operated, complained of disturbing instability. This and the enthusiasm initiated, by the hip arthroplasty, on the one hand, and our disappointment with our use of the condyle-sacrificing prosthesis from Swanson and McKee, on the other, induced us to develop a prosthesis which could be inserted between the humerus condyles and cemented in with stems in the humerus and ulna. Consistent with a constrained hinge, the axis was rigidly mounted; the movement being transmitted to the ulna by way of a ring free to swivel but attached to the humerus component. A screw working in accordance with the double cone principle bound both parts tightly together. To what extent we placed our trust in the intercondylar position of the prosthesis and the retained, remaining condyles, and the ligaments and muscles, is reflected by the very thin stems. To increase the rotational stability and to allow the operation of cases where the humerus had been resected as a result of a previous operation (resection arthroplasty, state after implantation of other prosthesis, traumatic loss of the condyles), we subsequently lengthened and bent the stems and provided them with rotation-stabilizing fins. (Fig. 1) Six years after implantation of the first prosthesis, the results are as follows.(Tab. 1 - 6)

The increase in movement is very satisfactory. In the majority of cases, the patients suffered no significant pain. However, the high proportion of loose prostheses was disturbing, this was evident in twelve of the first thirty-nine cases four years after implantation. Even if we allow for the fact that in five cases other forms of arthroplasty, which had sacrificed the condyles, had preceded the implantation of our GSB prosthesis and the more frequent consumption of steroids provide a valid explanation for cases of loosening, there is no doubt that our intercondylar, minimal resecting, constrained-hinge prosthesis had not fulfilled expectations. The circumstance that the complaints made by the majority of patients with loosened prostheses were only trivial, and the removal of the prosthesis enabled a remarkably stable and well movable simple resection arthroplasty to be realized (Fig. 2) are insufficient reasons for us to adhere to our initial model. This is still true even though the very first patient, who was operated on 6 years ago, still has a painless and extensive range of motion and no signs of loosening! (Fig. 3)

When we analyse the causes of loosening, three types of forces may be considered responsible:

1. Forces acting on the fully extended arm: On lifting a weight, the anchorage of the prosthesis in the humeral shaft and in the ulna experiences a pull corresponding approximately to the weight lifted. This stress will be reduced by the pull of the muscles crossing the elbow, having always a certain tone even at rest. As the artificial elbows are rarely held in a fully extended position, we have to consider the situation during flexion. According to Pauwels the force relationship of the flexors of the upper arm to the forearm flexors is 3:5. Both muscle groups run in extension nearly parallel to the arm. During contraction they exhibit a considerable axial force amounting about to ten times the load lifted. In praxis this means that carrying a weight exhibits first a pull on the prosthesis, and then the cement. The resulting compression reaches about 200 kp. A similar situation occurs, when leaning with the hand upon a table or using crutches. In such a situation the body weight and

the pull of the extensors, trying to counteract a giving-way of the elbow has to be added. The ulnar stem becomes a one arm leverarm, with its fulcrum on the lower end, which presses on the posterior ulnar wall. This leverage is particularly high, when lifting an object to a higher level (eg. a tray).
The frequently changing compression and pulling power may, particularly in a osteoporotic bone, be responsible for the 'sinking-in' of the prosthesis mainly in the humerus, as well as for some spontaneous fractures on the weakend humeral condyle. Here we have also to consider forces, which we will discuss later.

2. At least equal importance has to be attributed to the forces acting on the flexed elbow. The resultant force runs from below-distally upwards and amounts to ten times the lifted weight. As it runs nearly parallel to the ulna, the distal stem undergoes only compression forces. But, the joint itself is pushed firmly backwards producing a pressure peak at the posterior wall on the distal humrus. As we have now a two-arm lever, the proximal end of the humeral stem will be pressed against the anterior wall of the humerus. The relationship of the moment arm being 1:5, it results in a compression force of 240 kp on the posterior humeral wall and 40 kp on the stem-end. (Fig. 4) Whereas in a normal elbow joint this force is transmitted mostly to the capitulum of the humerus and only a relatively small force component to the ulnar trochles, (Fig. 5) in all artificial joint the resection of the radial head must necessarily transmit these forces to the previously mentioned points of anchorage of the prosthesis in the humerus. The following X-rays may give the proof of the correctness of this assumption (Fig.6). The prosthesis is pushed backwards and the humeral stem has perforated the anterior wall. You may compare the stem-position in extension and in flexion. Another proof for this kind of mechanism is shown in this simple resection arthroplasty, which I performed years ago. The sling-like action of the forearmflexors pulls the humerus foreward on the ulna and it is only during further flexion that the muscle-pull is diminished and the humerus glides again backwards on the ulna. See the X-rays of the patient. (Fig. 7)

3. Finally let us consider the rotational stresses on the forearm during pro- and supi-nation. As the radial head has been resected, there is necessarily an increased rotation stress on the ulna. Since the ratio of the radius of the distal radio-ulnar junction to the ulnar-stem-radius being about 10:1, the additional possibility of this stem getting loose arises. (Fig. 8) Much more importance has to be attributed to the forces arising during rotation of the arm, when pushing objects on a table aside or - even worse -

when lifting objects with the abducted arm. The axis of rotation runs through the humerus, will be transmitted to the humeral stem and via the artificial joint to the forearm. The relationship of the leverarm, corresponding to the lengths of the forearm, to the radius of the stem, is in the old GSB model 100:1,(Fig. 9) it becomes evident, why much more loosenings occured in the humeral component.
We now also understand, why the application of an antirotational flange of the humeral stem in our second model, resulted in a loosening of the ulnar component.

On the basis of the statements made, one wonders what the prosthesis of the future will look like. In principle, there are two possibilities at our disposal:

1. A surface-type prosthesis which endeavours to imitate the articular faces in one way or another. For example the prosthesis of Ewald or of Engelbrecht. The various types may be differentiated through the mode of fixation (pure surface fixation, fixation by means of intracondylar or intramedular pins).

2. Composite prostheses, whose components are loosely connected with each other.

We have selected the second approach for our new GSB-joint, (Fig. 10) because

1. The surface-type prosthesis can dislocate, especially if the muscles and ligaments are poor.

2. With greater alteration of the anatomical conditions (e.g. intraarticular fractures), it may be technically very difficult to apply a surface-type prosthesis.

The differences between the new and old GSB prosthesis are as follows:

1. The new model rests with a broad bearing surface on the humerus condyles and can thus take up practically all the forces acting from the distal to proximal and ventral to dorsal direction.

2. The connection between the humeral and ulnar components is a loose one, allowing a play of 4° to 5° of the ulnar component in the swivelable, polyethylene-coated ring of the humerus component.

3. The stems are stronger and better suited to the medullary canal than was the case with the old version.

The operation technique is the same, apart from the fact that the condyles have to be rounded off with a spherical burr to such an extent that they are able to be gripped well by the prosthesis.

The value of this new design cannot be assessed so far because of the absence of significant clinical experience. Nevertheless, I should like to show you the pre- and post-operative radiological and clinical picture of the first case provided with the new prosthesis.(Fig.11a-c)

The GSB wrist-joint

Without doubt, the wrist joint is one of the most complicated joints in the human body. Apart from the positive experience gathered in the majority of cases with arthrodesis, this will explain why we have not been satisfied so far with either the simple resection arthroplasty or artificial joints that only permit a flexion-extension or the ball and socket joint designs, which could not prevent with any certainty the rotation normally lacking in the wrist joint (admittedly, the absence of actual wrist-joint rotation muscles, respectively the small lever arm of the ab/adducting muscles in respect of rotation does not appear to be of any great significance). In our efforts to obtain the best possible physiological extent of movement and, simultaneously, good stability, we arrived at the following design principle (Fig. 12):

A ball with two protuding pins moving in a corresponding two-part hollow spherical housing. As a ball and socket joint, our prosthesis is only subject to one limitation of movement in the areas of movement which lie on the other side of the physiological movement range. It is only rotation that is rendered impossible by the lateral pins because, after all, it does not exist physiologically but takes place as pro/supination in the forearm. Instead, the GSB prosthesis permits a circumduction of the wrist joint which is a combination movement of dorso/palmar flexion and ab/adduction.

With the first generation, fixation was effected with a relatively thin stem in the Capitate and third metacarpal bone, respectively and the Radius by means of cement. We employed this prosthesis from 1971-73 and then stopped for further observation. The extent of bone resection (Fig. 13) is relatively small and, in the majority of cases, it relates only to one-half of the navicular bone, the Lunate and Triquetrum, the proximal half of the Capitate and the ulnar head. The degree to which the distal Radius has to be resected depends on the degree of any subluxation or dislocation.

Results
In the period from 1971 to 1975, we operated on 15 cases (Tab. 7). The indications consisted primarily of dislocated or subluxated painful polyarthritic wrist joints (Tab. 8) (Fig. 14) where a synovectomy or the simple resection of the distal ulnar end would have no longer shown any prospects of success and where arthrodesis was not considered owing to extensive destruction of the neighbouring joints. Relief from pain was realized in the majority of cases for the first two years after the

operation (Tab. 9).

The extent of movement (Fig. 15) was only slightly better post-operatively - a fact which is not surprising when one considers the severe pre-operative changes especially in regard to the massive musbular inbalance. The decisive factor, however, was the functionally substantial improvement in the range of movement towards dorsi flexion. Ab/adduction and circumduction movements were possible in the majority of cases. Whereas the value of the design principle would appear to be substantiated by these results, it was soon found that the fixation was completely inadequate and not matched in any way with the wrist joint loads. In 3 cases the distal stem became loose and in 2 cases the stem fractured (Fig. 16). On one occasion, the metacarpal bone broke at the same time (Fig. 17). During the subsequent arthrodesis, the wrist joint was fixed by means of a rush pin and rotation-stabilizing plate so that stable-exercises could be performed (Fig. 18). Thanks to the small amount of bone resection, it did not give rise to any special difficulties and was, in fact, successful. In another case, as a result of a disturbance of the muscle balance, we saw a fixed ulnar deviation of the wrist joint, with a tendency to radial penetration of the medullary canal of the third metacarpal bone. In 3 cases, we found a sinking of the prosthesis into the Capitate, through the third Metacarpal.

With the exception of 1 case, however, no loosening could be seen on the Radius.

New GSB wrist joint (Fig. 19)

Although the new GSB prosthesis is based on the same design of the joint itself, two distal stems now serve the anchorage in the Metacarpal II and III. Sinking and loosening are to be prevented in future by means of two wide supporting surfaces distally and proximally.

In this way, we hope to be able to extend the hitherto very restrictively applied indications to cases where, up to now, wrist arthrodesis was carried out primarily for reasons of safety. At the same time, we are quite aware of the necessity for an increased number of secondary operations in order to restore the frequently disturbed muscle balance by means of tendon transplantations.

In the case of arthroplasty of the MP-joint, the silastic prosthesis from Swanson rightfully dominates the field for the time being. The relative simplicity of the implantation, a low complication rate and good retreat possibilities definitely constitute valid arguments for its use. If work is proceeding on new prostheses in very different places, it is only because that we are all aware that the silastic implant is not a proper joint, but only a spacer which allows for better stability than the simple resection ar-

throplasty. More mobility, increased stability are the goals of all the latest designs. We are also endeavouring to implant prostheses without cement in order to reduce the possible consequences of an infectious complication to a minimum (Fig. 20). The joint section of the GSB prosthesis consists of two parts, which are connected together by a screw that serves simultaneously as the axis. A flexion of 100°, an over extension of 10° and a radial abduction - the extent of which decreases as flexion increases - permit a physiological function up to the intentionally blocked ulnar abduction. The fixation of the prosthesis is effected with screw-like cylinders made of Hostaform (a plastics material similar to polyester), which are available in seven different sizes and can be inserted in the bone after preparation of the bony bed. In addition, the slotted end of the cylinder is only prised about 1½ mm apart with a small wedge. Although the bones are now seated in the grooves of the screw thread, it would have resulted inevitably in loosening under the load of the daily activities, particularly with bones of inferior quality. Consequently, the prosthesis is now fixed in the plastic cylinder with a pin and in such a way that the prosthesis can slide to and fro in the event of pull on the fingers. This piston effect should stress the bone as little as possible. However, it is still too early to reach a verdict on the basis of the first 30 implanted joints.

At the level of the PIP joint, we have never been completely satisfied with the silastic prosthesis because of its insufficient stability. For the purpose of having a prosthesis which only necessitates a minimum of bone resection, is stable and exhibits a physiological scope of movement, we came to the following construction (Fig. 21). With its wide bearing articular surfaces, the proximal prosthesis part lies on the condyles of the phalanx head. It is sunk with the aid of a finned marrow space pin between the condyles. As a result, should an arthrodesis become necessary, we only have to contend with minimal shortening and, furthermore we have good spongy contact surfaces at our disposal. A similar wide bearing surface is in contact with the base of the central phalanx, where only about 1 mm of bone has to be ground away. The connection between these two prosthesis components is a loose one both in the proximal-distal, as well as in the lateral direction. Both parts are assembled under slight flexion. Although fixation can be effected with only a small amount of cement, we are hoping that the marrow space pins, thanks to their christmas tree-like profile with very rough surface of sintered metal, will soon be able to be anchored without any cement at all.

110

In Figure 22 we can see the first patient to be provided with this prosthesis. The indication showed a partly stiffened, very painful arthrosis. There are no more complaints, mobility is only restricted to a minimum degree. Here again, it is still too early to make any appraisal of this process.

To sum up, it may be stated in the case of GSB joints for the upper extremity that the principle of minimal resection has proven successful. Instead of the constrained hinged prosthesis, we will only have loosely connected ones in future. We feel that they offer the best guarantee for stable movement.

Table 1

GSB-Elbow-Arthroplasty 1971-1974

Implanted articulations	39
Age	40 years (25-63)
Time since operation	37 months (12-60)

Table 3

GSB-Elbow-Arthroplasty 1971-1974

PAIN	preoperative	postoperative
O	4	23
mild	2	14
medium	9	2
severe	24	O

Table 2

GSB-Elbow-Arthroplasty 1971-1974

MOBILITY

Flexion	preoperative	postoperative
more than 130	9	21
90 - 130	15	18
- 90	5	O
ankylosis	10	O

Table 4

Klinik Wilhelm Schulthess
Zürich 1975

GSB-Elbow-Arthroplasty n = 39

Complication - Loosening n = 12

3 developping spontaneous fracture lateral humeral condyle

5 developping spontaneous perforation of humeral shaft

Table 5

GSB-Elbow-Arthroplasty n = 39

Complication: Loosening n = 12

Model	first	10	last	2
Site	Humerus	7	Ulna	2
	both	3		

Time after surgery:	> 4 years	3	(7)
	3-4 years	5	(14)
	2-3 years	3	(8)
	< 2 years	1	(10)

Table 6

GSB-Elbow-Arthroplasty n = 39

Complication - Loosening n = 12

Concomitant factors

	No Loosening n = 27	Loosening n = 12
Previous operation	O	3
Using canes or crutches	12	7
No canes or crutches	15	5
Steroids	15	8

Table 7

GSB-Wrist-Arthroplasty

Patients operated		15
males	3	
females	12	
Age minimal	36	
maximal	68	
average		55
Hands		15
right	10	
left	5	

Table 8

GSB-Wrist-Arthroplasty

Indications

RA   15

with luxation or
       subluxation   12

with fixed flexion   3

Table 9

GSB-Wrist-Arthroplasty

| Results | | PAIN |
preoperative		postoperative
-	none	12
-	slight	3
7	moderate	-
8	severe	-

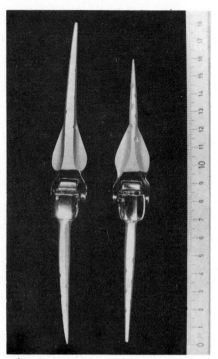

Fig. 1:

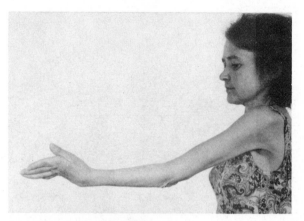

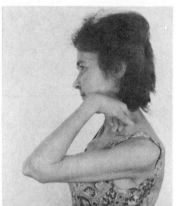

Fig. 2:

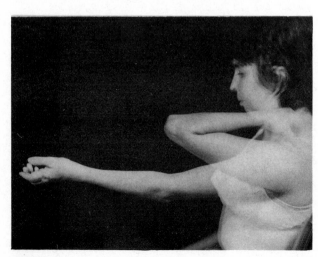

Fig. 3:

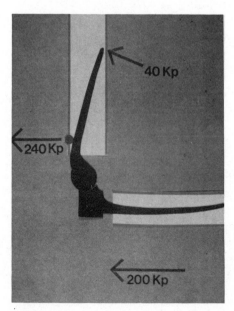

Fig. 4:

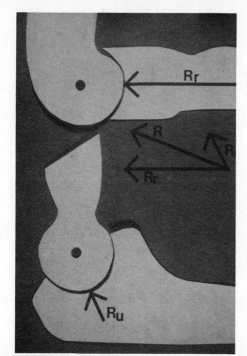

Fig. 5:

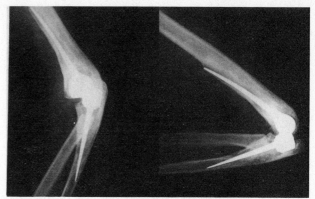

Fig. 6:

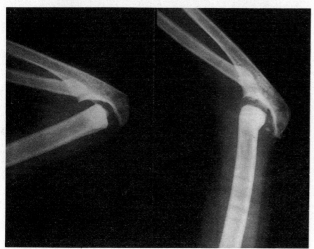

Fig. 7:

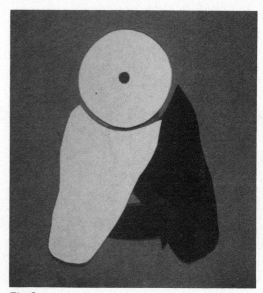

Fig. 8:

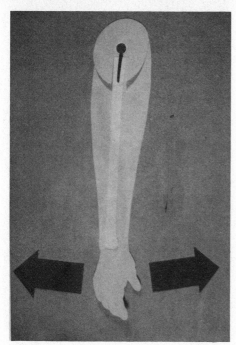

Fig. 9:

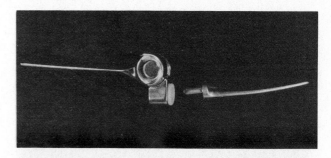

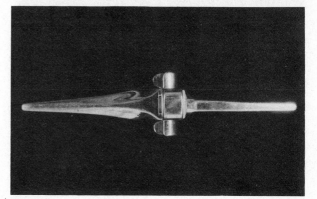

Fig. 10:

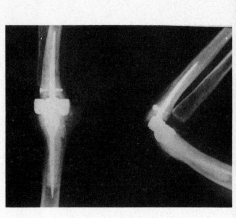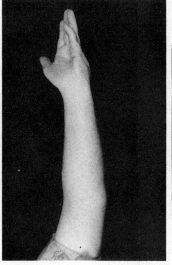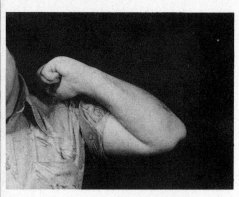

Fig. 11:

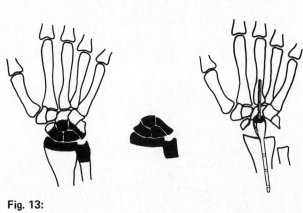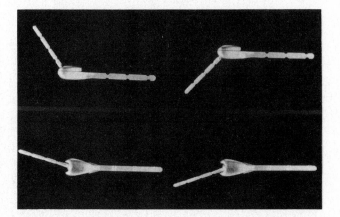

Fig. 12:

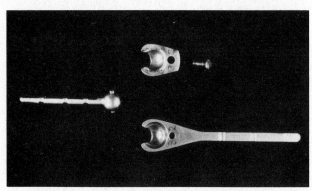

Fig. 13:

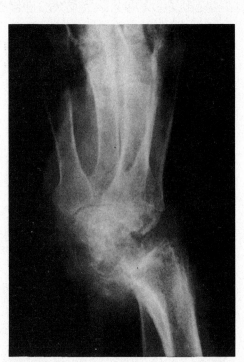

Fig. 14:

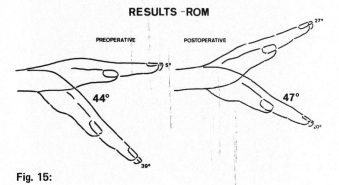

KLINIK WILHELM SCHULTHESS
Zürich

GSB - WRIST - ARTHROPLASTY

RESULTS - ROM

PREOPERATIVE   POSTOPERATIVE

27°

5°

44°   47°

20°

39°

Fig. 15:

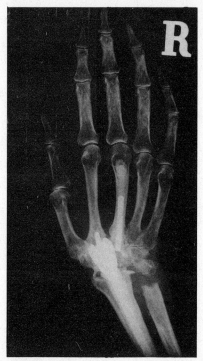

Fig. 16:

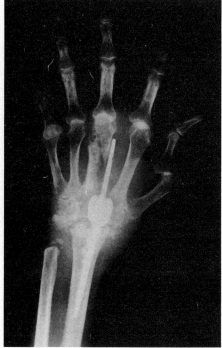

Fig. 17:

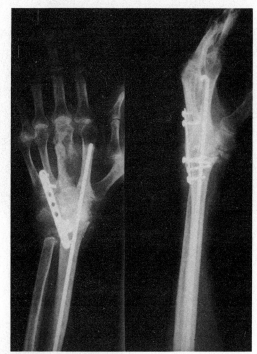

Fig. 18:

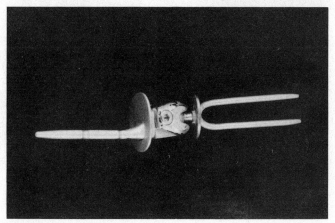

Fig. 19:

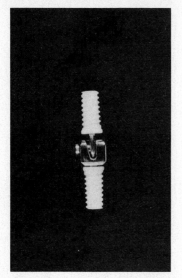

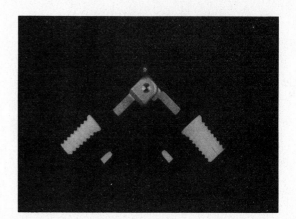

Fig. 20:

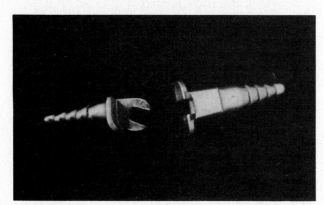

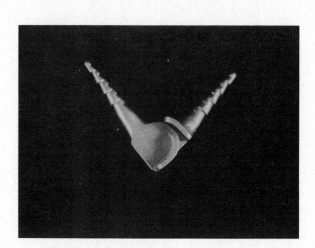

Fig. 21:

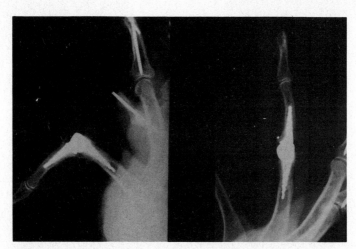

Fig. 22:

TOTAL WRIST JOINT REPLACEMENT

H. Ch. MEULI, MD,
University of Berne and Lindenhofspital Berne

SYNOPSIS   A new total wrist joint prosthesis is presented. The concept and the design of the prosthesis as well as the technique of the operation are described. The experience with the first 26 wrist
joint replacements after a follow up period of 5½ years is reported. The results permit this method to
be recommended for selected cases. Technical difficulties encountered at the beginning can now be controlled. If failure occurs, the prosthesis can be replaced, it is also possible, if needed, later to
perform an arthrodesis with bone grafting.

1. Introduction

In the last few years, alloplastic joint replacement has had an unprecedented upswing. Treatment
of hip osteoarthritis without total hip arthroplasty is unimaginable. Today replacement arthroplasty of many other joints is increasingly being
carried out. It was a logical consequence to consider replacement of the wrist joint. However,
this joint prosthesis is one of the last to be
developed. The reason for this might be that
arthrodesis of the wrist has been a reliable
method of treatment. Bony wrist fusion is suitable for young manual workers where a painless
wrist without loss of strength and with only in-
significant loss of function is desirable. The
first operations on the wrist joint were in the
19th century, when Kocher (1), Ollier (2), von
Langenbeck (3) and others performed wrist joint
resections. It seems that the German military
surgeon Beyer was the first to carry out wrist
joint resection arthroplasty during war time in
1762. Today the resection of the first row of
carpal bones with interposition of fascia lata is
still a 'classical' method of wrist arthroplasty
(Bunnell (4), Crabbe (5), Stamm (6)). Sometimes
the second row of carpal bones is resected as
well.

For some time now corrective osteotomies, partial
arthrodeses and partial arthroplasties have made
satisfactory functional reconstruction possible.
The introduction of flexible Silicone implants by
Swanson (7) was one of the most remarkable ad-
vances in joint replacement surgery. But the
existing arthroplasties could not guarantee
sufficient movement and were not completely satisfactory in regard to stability. The statement by
Bunnell (4) 'True arthroplasty is seldom indicated
in the wrist' might have been quite correct.

In surgery of rheumatoid arthritis especially in
the case of bilateral wrist joint destruction, in
older people or in women who do not do heavy work,
arthroplasty has found increasing application. We
have been engaged, for a number of years, in developing a total wrist joint replacement (Fig. 1).
This wrist joint prosthesis was published for the
first time at the annual spring meeting of the
French Association for Hand Surgery (GEM) in 1972

(8). Today we are able to report our clinical experience of the last 5½ years.

2. The Concept

In developing a wrist joint prosthesis the following criteria were decisive:

From the beginning it was obvious that only a
simple construction could guarantee a good function. The employment of materials with adequate
mechanical properties was self evident. We pro-
fited from the experiences in developing other
joint prostheses. The physiological joint movement had to be imitated as closely as possible.
Impingement of components of the joint had to be
avoided because of the danger of loosening. Stability was necessary to enable the arthritic
patient to use a cane. Finally, a salvage procedure had to be possible. For this reason extensive bone resection was not desirable since
bony fusion would not be possible.

All these considerations finally led to the development of a ball joint. Although the wrist
joint is, in reality, much more complicated, consisting of several individual joints, the total
function of the wrist, however, corresponds to
that of a ball joint with a constant axis of
motion located on the capitate.

The prosthesis (Fig. 2) manufactured by Sulzer
Brothers Limited in Winterthur, consists of three
parts: a metallic stem which is placed into the
radius and a metallic cup which is placed into the
metacarpals II and III (IV). Between both parts a
polyethylene ball is interposed. This construction assures free movement in several directions.
Besides flexion and extension, radial and ulnar
abduction, a rotational movement and a certain
degree of distraction is possible. We assume that
through this system stresses and strains are more
equally distributed. Both metal parts are made of
Protasul 10 and have two prongs which are anchored in bone using bone cement . This type of fixation enables a better adaption of the prosthesis
to the elasticity of the bone. Additionally the
spikes can be individually bent permitting an exact centering of the prosthesis.

Different prototypes were necessary until the prosthesis evolved to its present form. While earlier
models were somewhat cumbersome it became possible
to reduce the size of the prongs. As experience
showed that luxation was not to be feared the cup
was made flatter. This enabled the range of
motion to be increased to 140° in all directions.

At the same time as the prosthesis, several special instruments were developed (Fig. 3). Two
bending irons to adjust the prongs of the prosthesis are indispensable. Otherwise the usual
hand surgery instruments are used.

3. The technique of the operation

Preoperative planning is indispensable. The anteroposterior and lateral radiographs of the wrist
are carefully studied. With the help of templates
and the radiographs the position and size of the
prosthesis is determined. For the operation one
should have both sizes of prosthesis and of polyethylene balls available. Sterilization of polyethylene can not be carried out in the operating
theatre. All the usual instruments used in hand
surgery should be at hand, as well as a small
drilling machine and a small oscillating saw.

The patient lies supine, the arm and hand are
supported on a table. The procedure is carried
out under pneumatic tourniquet control. The operative field (hand and wrist) is covered with an
adhesive plastic film. The procedure is carried
out through a straight dorsal incision which
crosses the wrist joint obliquely from a disto-
radial in a proximo-ulnar direction. The extensor
retinaculum is carefully dissected out by detaching it from the ulnar side and preserving its
radial attachment. The extensor tendons are then
retracted which exposes the wrist joint. The bones
to be excised are: the scaphoid, the lunate, the
proximal half of the capitate and the articular
part of the radius (Fig. 4). A synovectomy, if
necessary, is carried out and a volar capsulotomy
or capsulectomy is completed. Anchor holes in the
radius and in the shafts of the metacarpals are
prepared using the awl and rasps. If necessary, a
radiograph is taken for guidance. Either the large
or the small model is selected. The spikes of the
prosthesis are 'set' with the bending irons (Fig.
3 and 5) to fit the metacarpals, usually the second and
the third, but on occasion the second and the
fourth or the third and the fourth. Be sure to
bend the prongs 5 - 10° dorsally to ensure dors-
iflexion (Fig. 6a and 6b). The fit of the prosthetic components is tested. All ulnar and palmar
tendons (e.g. the flexor digitorum profundus,
the flexor carpi ulnaris) must be completely freed
up so that they can be made to glide freely. The
tendon tension must be accurately adjusted. The
tension must be moderate and balanced. Beware of
imbalance with one side in too much tension and
beware of tight prosthesis. Remember that under
anaesthesia all tendons are relaxed. The components are cemented in, beginning with the distal
one. The tourniquet is released and hemostatis is
secured. The artificial joint is assembled and
reduced. The components are then covered by passing the extensor retinaculum deep to the extensor
tendons and attaching it with a few interrupted
sutures. One deep suction drain is inserted to
drain the joint and another subcutaneously. A
padded dressing with a dorsal plaster slab for
support is applied.

4. The post-operative care

Begin with finger movements as well as exercises
for the elbow and shoulder. Remove the suction
drains in 48 hours and the initial dressing after
four days. Increase gradually the mobilization
of the joints. Unrestricted movement and increased function should begin after the first
three weeks. If extensor weakness is present, use
dynamic extensor support for some more weeks.

5. The results

Since 1971 we have performed 26 total endoprostheses of the wrist joint. This is a modest number of cases, when we realize that since 1974 in
the Mayo Clinic, more than 50 total wrist replacements using this prosthesis have been carried out
(R. D. Beckenbaugh and R. L. Linscheid (9)). We
have not published our results, in order to gain
more clinical experience and to learn how to control various complications. We considered it important to await the 5½ year results before recom-
mending the method for routine use.

Since 1971 21 patients, 15 females, 6 males have
had the operation, this includes both wrists in
three patients. Twice the prosthesis has been
changed. 1 Patient has since died. Indication
for the operation has been rheumatoid arthritis
in 20 cases and post traumatic osteoarthritis in
4 cases. Questioning of the 21 patients has
shown that 18 are satisfied and 3 dissatisfied.
The postoperative evaluation gave 9 unsatisfactory
primary results. In 6 cases a satisfactory result was obtained after reoperation. The maximal
follow up period was 5½ years.

Fig. 7 shows radiographs of a patient
during a four year period. Obviously we have had
several failures (Table 1). This was not unex-
pected considering that this was a new untried
method. In spite of this we could control most
complications so that the majority of patients
finally were very pleased with the result. Infection, the most important and feared complication, occured in two cases. In one case with
severe rheumatoid arthritis the operation was performed under unfavourable surgical conditions.
After removal of the prosthesis a successful arthrodesis with a bone graft was carried out. In a
second case, the diagnosis of tuberculosis of the
bone was made histologically only after removal of
the prosthesis. In this case it was also possible
to achieve successful bony fusion using a bone
graft. As has been the experience of other groups,
we have had difficulties with the ulnar deviation
which occurs if the prosthesis is not exactly
centred. The bending irons permit us to individually center the cup. Additionally the tendon
tension must be balanced, it must not be too tense
and above all not one-sided. Perhaps, in time,
loosening of the prosthesis will be troublesome,
presently it is not. The construction of the
prosthesis for the significantly different and reduced forces of the wrist, compared for example
with the hip, should be adequate. However, the
observation time is still too short.

Unfortunately the first prototypes used polyester
as a material for the ball. This caused a severe
synovitis in several patients which led twice to
replacement of the prosthesis.

This operation is astonishingly simple. In one case a complete prosthesis change was necessary because loosening was suspected. The radiograph findings could not be confirmed clinically. In another case the prosthesis was replaced from a palmar approach simultaneously with a synovectomy of the carpal tunnel.

Following the evaluation of the functional results we have refrained from stating the exact range of motion. Also we do not consider the amount of strength as indicative of a good or poor result. The patient wishes above all a painless wrist. Although motion is usually very good, occasionally partial ankylosis has been observed. With good function and position of the hand movement of only a few degrees is useful. Strength must be sufficient for daily activities and suffice for the use of a cane. This has been achieved in all patients.

6. Conclusion and summary

The main indication for a total wrist arthroplasty is rheumatoid arthritis, particularly when both wrists are afflicted. A spontaneous fused painless wrist should not be replaced with a prosthesis. Usually excision of the distal end of the ulna is adequate to improve rotational movement. In the case of advanced malposition a tendon transfer combined with an arthroplasty is to be considered. The prosthesis should not be used if there is insufficiency of the extensor tendons. In cases of post traumatic arthrosis of the wrist, the total wrist arthroplasty is to be used with restraint. For most of these cases the treatment of choice is still an arthrodesis in a good functional position.

The results of 5½ years of clinical trial with total wrist arthroplasty permits this method to be recommended for selected cases. Technical difficulties encountered at the beginning can now be controlled. On failure the prosthesis can be replaced; it is also possible, if needed, later to perform an arthrodesis with bone grafting.

References:

(1) Kocher Th. (1897): Chirurgische Operationslehre. 3. Auflage, Jena, Verlag von Gustav Fischer.

(2) Ollier L. (1869): Des résections des grandes articulations. Lyon 8 (s. 23).

(3) von Langenbeck B. (1874): Chirurgische Beobachtungen aus dem Kriege, Berlin, Verlag von August Hirschwald.

(4) Bunnell S. (1964): Surgery of the Hand. 4th edition, revised by J. H. Boyes, Lippincott, Philadelphia.

(5) Crabbe W. A. (1961): Excision of the proximal Row of the Carpus. J. Bone Jt Surg. 46 B.

(6) Stamm T. T. (1944): Excision of the proximal Row of the Carpus, Proc. roy. Soc. Med. (Sect. of orthopaedics), 38, 74.

(7) Swanson A. B. (1973): Flexible implant resection arthroplasty in the hand and extremities, The C. V. Mosby Company St. Louis.

(8) Meuli H. Ch. (1973): Arthroplastie du poignet, Ann. Chir. 27, 15, pp. C 527-530.

(9) Beckenbaugh R. D. and Linscheid R. L. (1976): personal communication.

TABLE I

COMPLICATIONS		REOPERATIONS	
1	INFECTION	1	ARTHRODESIS
1	TBC	1	ARTHRODESIS
2	ANKYLOSES IN MALPOSITION	1	ARTHRODESIS
		1	SOFT TISSUE RELEASE
1	ANKYLOSIS	1	REVISION, RESECTION RADIUS
1	ANKYLOSIS	Ø	
2	RECIDIVANT SYNOVITIS (POLYESTER)	2	SYNOVECTOMIES AND CHANGE OF PROSTHESES
1	LOOSENING	1	CHANGE OF PROSTHESIS PREVIEWED

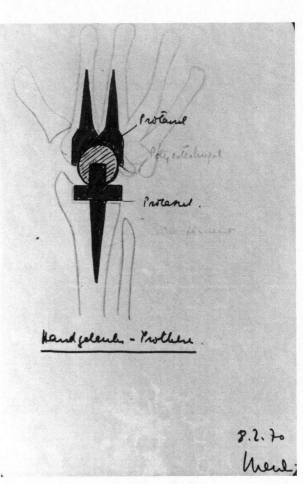

Fig. 1: First sketch of a wrist joint prosthesis

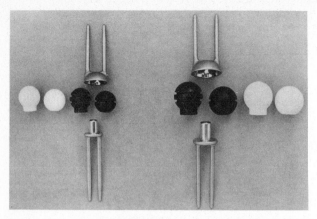

Fig. 2: The wrist joint prosthesis (with black test balls)

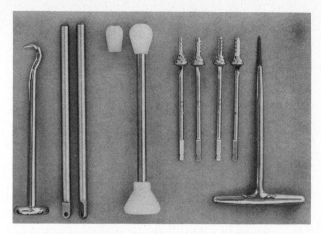

Fig. 3: The special instruments: awl, rasps, introducer, bending irons, extractor

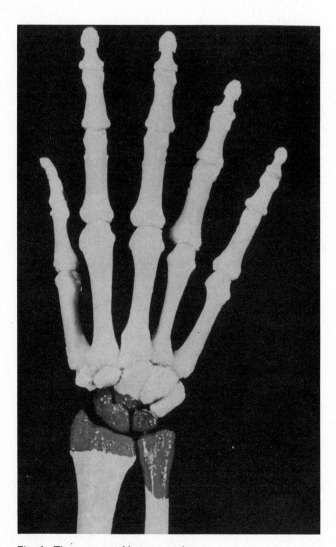

Fig. 4: The amount of bone resection

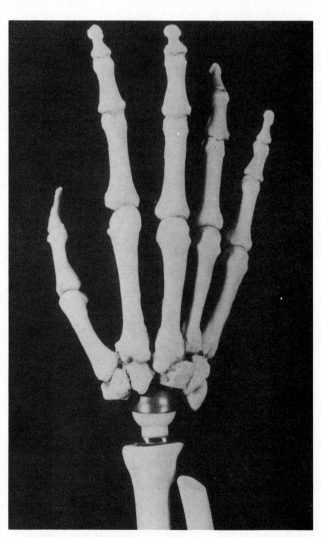

120

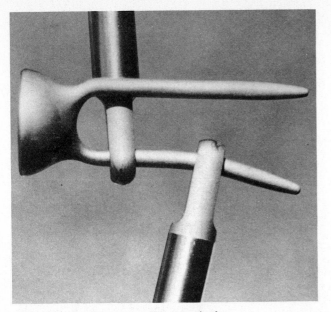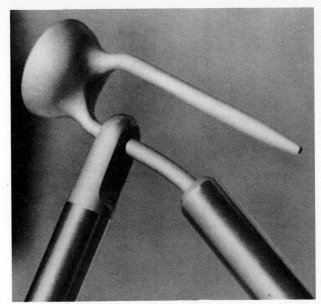

Fig. 5: Bending the prongs of the prosthesis

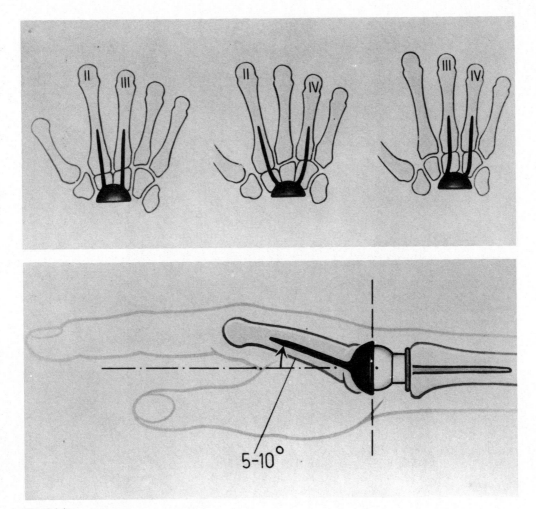

Fig. 6 (a):
     (b):   The positioning of the cup

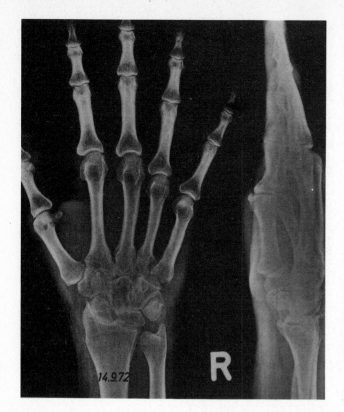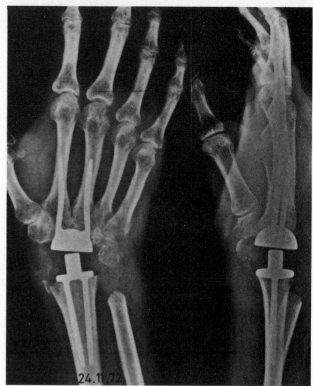
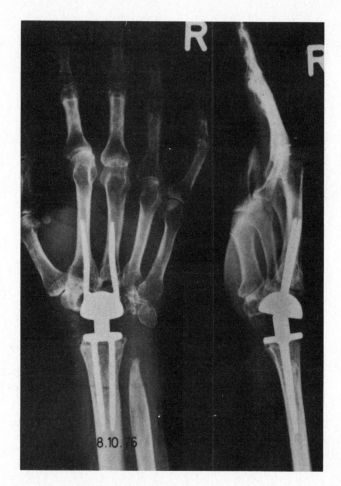

Fig. 7 (a): X-ray before operation
        (b): X-ray after operation
        (c): X-ray 4 years later — shows no changes

JOINT REPLACEMENT IN THE UPPER LIMB

C. G. ATTENBOROUGH, MChir, FRCS,
Royal East Sussex Hospital, Hastings

1. The stabilized gliding knee prosthesis was described at the Conference on Total Knee Replacement at the Institution of Mechanical Engineers in September 1974. This implant was designed as a compromise to give the stability which is lacking in surface prostheses but with sufficient designed rotational and lateral laxity to try to avoid the loosening which so frequently occurs with constrained hinge joints. Clinical trials started in January 1973, and by September 1976 more than 160 knees had been operated upon using this prosthesis at Hastings and 700 or 800 were in use throughout the world.

2. In a review of one and two year results of the first 160 knees operated on in Hastings satisfactory results have been achieved even where there has been a pre-existing severe deformity or ligamentous laxity and there has been no case of spontaneous loosening of a component.

3. Some of the problems of the knee are the same as those in some joints in the upper limb, notably the elbow. The ligaments of the elbow are often damaged to an even greater degree than the knee joint and constrained hinged joints in the elbow are subject to loosening as much as, if not more than in the knee joint. It seemed reasonable, therefore, to try to design an elbow joint on the stabilized gliding principle which appears to be successful in the knee. It must be remembered that in the joints of the upper limb the weight-bearing loads are usually absent and the compression force is from muscle activity only. There is, however, in marked contrast to the joints of the lower limb, a considerable distraction force. This is present most of the time from the weight of the limb but must rise significantly in certain actions when carrying a weight or endeavouring to pull an object. It is probable that in the normal elbow joint much of this distraction force is carried by the ligaments but if these are seriously damaged then the joint itself will have to take the distraction load. In such circumstances a totally unconnected surface prosthesis will run the danger of dislocation and a totally

constrained hinge will have this distraction force to cause loosening, in addition to the rotational strains.

4. The stabilized gliding elbow joint (Fig. 1) consists of humeral and ulnar components, stabilized by a rod similar to that in the knee joint prosthesis and allowing gliding flexion and extension with rotational and lateral laxity which are controlled partly by the stabilizing rod itself and partly by the designed opening of the joint when it rotates or when lateral strains are applied. In these circumstances the remaining soft tissues tend to tighten and help to produce a gradual deceleration of rotation or lateral movement rather than a sudden stop.

5. The humeral component is made in chrome cobalt alloy. It has two hollowed condyles which fit over the lower end of the humerus and a tapered intramedullary stem with rounded corners. Between the condylar runners is a groove into which fits a high density polyethylene component which is in two parts (Fig. 2). Each part snaps into the metal humeral component in the manner of a circlip and the two parts when in position enclose the ball of the stabilizing rod (Figs. 3, 4 and 5). The high density polyethylene components are relatively easily inserted but once in position can only be removed with great difficulty, except by destruction with a drill. The components are so shaped that the stabilizing rod can move into a position of full flexion and extension, allowing a little lateral movement. In all positions the stabilizing rod is kept from touching the metal humeral component itself.

6. The humeral runners have a two radii curve, the longer radius being in front and behind and the smaller radius distally. The ulnar component made in high density polyethylene has a tapered intramedullary stem of the same dimensions as that of the humeral component. The proximal end of this component consists of a plateau which is set at 30 degrees to the angle of the stem. Each side of this plateau is hollowed to fit exactly the longer

anterior and posterior curves of the humeral runners. Between the two sides of the plateau there is a hole into which fits the stabilizing rod and either side of this a hole of smaller diameter which runs to the bottom of the central hole and should prevent the build up of any pressure beyond the stabilizing rod. As in the knee joint, this stabilizing rod moves within the distal component because of the two different curves of the humeral component. This may help to lubricate the joint and the stabilizing rod itself.

7.   When the joint is fully extended or fully flexed, the two components fit exactly and there is good rotational stability but the joint will allow some rotation if the strain is severe. As it rotates, the joint opens tightening the soft tissues. When the joint is semi-flexed the shorter radius of the humeral component is in contact with the now larger radius of the ulnar component and rotation is freer but the joint still opens tightening the soft tissues, as before. The stabilizing rod allows some lateral movement but controls this in a gradual fashion as the movement is centred around one or other condyle and not round both the condyles together. Once again then the joint tends to open when a lateral strain is applied tightening the soft tissues. The stabilizing rod also allows the two components to distract without danger of dislocation.

OPERATIVE TECHNIQUE

8.   The implant is inserted through a posterior approach. The skin incision starts in the midline over the triceps, curves towards the inner side over the' medial post condylar groove and then curves back to the midline over the shaft of the ulna. The incision is deepened to the deep fascia and the ulnar nerve is identified, mobilized and gently retracted medially. The triceps muscle and tendon are split in the midline down to the olecranon and then cut from the olecranon by sharp dissection, and further distally the periosteum is stripped from the upper end of the ulna for a distance of about 5 centimetres. This leaves the triceps in continuity with the periosteum of the ulna. The joint is opened in the same line by dividing the capsule and synovial membrane and the exposure is increased by stripping the capsule gently from the lower end of the humerus until the whole of the articular surface of the humerus and ulna are visible. The head of the radius is excised just distal to the groove on the ulna. The olecranon is excised with an oscillating saw directing the blade distally so that the angle of the cut is at 30 degrees to the longitudinal axis of the ulna with the distal cut finishing at the level of the base of the coracoid process.

9.   About 1 centimetre of bone is removed from the lower end of the humerus with an oscillating saw. This cut must be at right angles to the axis of the humerus in both planes. The anterior surface of the lower end of the humerus may also need to be trimmed so that the antero-posterior thickness will fit within the condyles of the humeral component. The posterior surface is left untouched in order to try to preserve the integrity of the humeral condyles. Occasionally some osteophytes may also need to be trimmed. A slot is cut in the lower end of the humerus wide enough to accommodate the central part of the humeral component and extending proximally as far as the olecranon notch. The medullary cavity of the humerus above the olecranon notch is opened using nibbling forceps, and a blunt ended guidewire is passed up the shaft of the humerus within the medullary cavity. A canulated tapered reamer is used to enlarge the medullary cavity to fit the stem of the humeral component. The medullary cavity of the ulna is enlarged in the same way, using the same guidewire and reamer.

10.   The reamer is designed to enlarge the medullary cavity so that the diameter is a few millimetres larger than the stem of the prosthesis and the depth a few millimetres longer than the length of the stem.

11.   One half of the high density polyethylene plug is inserted into the humeral component and a trial fit is undertaken linking the two components but not inserting the second high density polyethylene plug. If full extension cannot be obtained, it may be necessary to trim a little more bone length from the humerus. Once a satisfactory range of movement has been obtained, the components are removed and cement introduced into the ulna, using a disposable bladder syringe with a special screw attachment fitted to the barrel. This is necessary as it is almost impossible to drive the barrel of the syringe in by hand alone. The ulnar component is then inserted. Cement is then introduced into the humerus and the humeral component inserted with the high density polyethylene component anterior. Once the cement is hard, the ulnar and humeral components are brought into apposition and the stabilizing rod inserted into the ulnar component, the ball engaging against the high density polyethylene plug already in the humeral component. The second half of the high density polyethylene plug is inserted so that the ball of the stabilizing rod is now captive within the humeral component (Figs. 3, 4 and 5).

12.   The wound is closed in layers with one suction drain in the joint and one in the subcutaneous tissues. A light pressure dressing is applied with the elbow at right angles.

POST-OPERATIVE CARE

13. Gentle active movements are permitted from the start. The pressure dressing and suction drainage tubes are removed after 48 hours and the patients continue to use a sling for as long as they find it necessary. Some of them have discarded it within a week. Most of the patients regain their movements with minimal supervised physiotherapy.

14. Clinical trials of this prosthesis only started in 1976 and it is much too early to assess the results, particularly as the failure of the cement-bone bond in hinged elbow prostheses often occurs between one and two years from the time of operation. Assessment of the clinical results of this prosthesis must, therefore, be delayed for at least two years. The initial range of movement obtained has been encouraging and the relatively easy rotation within the prosthesis can be felt. It is hoped this will act as a safety mechanism to avoid the breakdown of the cement-bone interface. This rather free rotation is well controlled by the patients who are able to lift quite heavy objects such as kettles and saucepans with the elbow flexed to a right angle, which necessarily incurs a considerable rotational strain.

WRIST AND HAND.

15. The stabilized gliding principle has also been applied to the wrist and to the metacarpophalangeal joints of the hand.

The Wrist.

16. Arthrodesis of the wrist gives an excellent clinical and functional result but arthrodesis of both wrists, particularly in elderly arthritic patients can be a severe disability. There is, therefore, probably a place for a total wrist replacement prosthesis. Such a prosthesis must allow the normal flexion, extension, ulnar and radial deviation of the wrist but rotation does not occur at the wrist joint. Most wrist implants so far designed have been of the ball and socket type, allowing rotation to occur freely in the wrist joint itself, whereas in the normal wrist the carpus rotates with the radius and rotation is, in fact, occurring at the elbow joint. If, however, there is total restraint of rotation at the wrist joint level, there will be a strain on the cement-bone interface both at the lower end of the radius and at the distal fixation of the wrist implant. The stabilized gliding principle has been applied, therefore, to produce an implant for the wrist joint with semi-constraint of rotation and still allowing distraction.

17. Distal fixation into the metacarpals has also to be carefully considered because there is differential movement between the metacarpals in most cases, although in some instances this may already have been prevented by damage from rheumatoid disease. If differential movement still remains, then fixed stems into the two metacarpals will inevitably produce a strain on the cement-bone bond. In the stabilized gliding wrist joint differential movement has been allowed to occur between the stems in order to try to overcome this problem.

Clinical trials of this prosthesis are due to commence early in 1977.

Metacarpophalangeal Joints.

18. A prosthesis has been made for use in the metacarpophalangeal joints. As well as flexion to a right angle, this prosthesis allows free rotation and limited lateral movement. If lateral movement is allowed to be completely free then it is impossible to control ulnar drift. So far this prosthesis has only been used in four instances and it has been found that the degree of torsional strain which a patient applies to the metacarpophalangeal joint with the joint flexed is such that the cement-bone bond has failed in the metacarpal in all instances. The patients themselves have achieved a good range of movement and have no pain and are happy with their prostheses but they are, nevertheless, technical failures. It seems probable that cement will never be a satisfactory method of fixing prostheses in the distal metacarpal shaft or the proximal phalanges and if this particular prosthesis is to be used again, it will have to be with some other form of fixation.

19. The results of coated prostheses are awaited with interest.

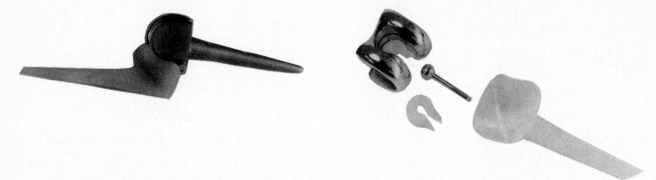

Fig. 1: The stabilized gliding elbow prosthesis assembled

Fig. 2: The separated components

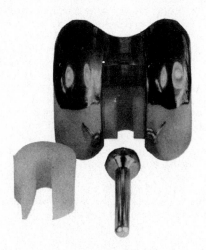

Fig. 3: One half of the high density polyethylene plug inserted

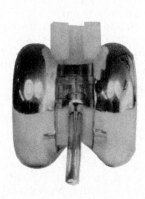

Fig. 4: The stabilizing rod in position

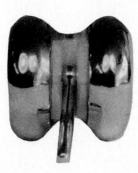

Fig. 5: The completed assembly with the stabilizing rod and
ball captive

DEVELOPMENT AND EVALUATION OF A MECHANICAL FINGER PROSTHESIS

P. S. WALKER, PhD, CEng, MIMechE
Codman & Shurtleff, Inc., Randolph, Mass.02368, USA
L. R. STRAUB, MD, W. DAVIDSON, MD, M. S. MONEIM, MD
Hospital for Special Surgery, New York, NY10021, USA

SYNOPSIS The earliest mechanical metacarpophalangeal joint prostheses were the metallic hinges of Brannon & Klein, and of F. R. Thompson, later modified by Flatt. The main problems were erosion of the stems through the bone, and fracture of the stems due to fatigue. Flatt and associates subsequently showed the importance of the correct biomechanics to prosthetic replacement. The silicone rubber spacer devised by Swanson has been used extensively over about the past ten years, with considerable success. Niebauer's design also utilises silicone rubber. However, fracture of the stem, inadequate range of motion and limited strength, have occurred in a sufficient percentage of patients in these silicone rubber prostheses to justify research into improved designs. One of the earliest mechanical designs utilising metal-plastic was the St. Georg. The two components popped together and considerable laxity was built in. Range of motion in the patient was often limited, apparently due to the ingress of fibrous tissue into the joint. The Steffee finger was another early metal-plastic design, again using a pop-in system. In a recent follow-up at the Mayo Clinic of 411 joints from 2 - 28 months, the average active range of motion was about 45° but the grip strength was not improved after operation. (Ref. 1). There was residual mild-moderate ulnar drift in nearly half of the cases.
2.   Whatever prosthesis is used, the result is limited by the state of the muscles and ligaments. However, a silicone rubber spacer has a limited capacity to accept shear forces and bending moments, while the mechanical designs have the potential to obtain a stronger result. The purpose of this paper is to report our experience in determining the optimum design parameters for such a prosthesis.

STUDIES OF THE NORMAL MCP JOINT

1. The morphology and motion of joint specimens were studied (Ref. 2). The metacarpal head and the phalangeal surface approximated to spherical surfaces, agreeing with other studies.(Ref. 3,4) In the lateral plane, the angle of enclosure of the phalanx was 60°, implying that shear forces of up to 60% of the compressive force could be sustained. In the a-p plane the bone sections were symmetrical.

In the lateral plane, the medullary canals were trumpet shaped, converging towards the centre, diverging again in the metacarpal and remaining parallel in the phalanx. The internal bone surfaces displayed 1/2mm ripples. The sections were non-circular, triangular in the metacarpal, and semicircular in the phalanx. These various features are advantageous to cement fixation in pull-out and in rotation. The centre of the metacarpal ball was below the centre-line of the shaft. The centre of rotation in flexion-extension on specimens varied with the angle of flexion and did not coincide with the geometrical centre. On average, the centre of rotation was 2mm distal and 1mm dorsal, in relation to the geometrical centre.

MECHANICAL EVALUATION OF THE NORMAL AND ARTHRITIC HAND

1. In evaluating a new prosthesis for the finger, particularly when improved function is one of the specific aims, it is important to be able to measure function objectively. There have been several reports on the use of instruments for measuring strength, motion and manipulative ability, including the application to prosthetic replacement. (Ref. 5,6,7) Our objective was to devise a comprehensive test which would cover all of these

aspects and be completed in a short period of time. The apparatus is shown in Figure 1. Active and passive motion were measured at 0° and at 60° of flexion. The various strengths were measured using strain-gauged beams, the output being on a digital recorder. Pulp pinch, lateral pinch, key pinch and chuck pinch were measured. The radial and ulnar forces exerted by the fingers were determined. For grip strength, a 37mm diameter tube was used, the outer layer being of sponge rubber. To measure manipulative ability, the time was taken to move four pegs requiring different turning and placing actions, from one set of holes to another.
2. Eighty normal females and 60 normal males, with ages ranging from 17 to 70 years were tested. In addition, thirty pre-operative female patients, most in their sixties with severe rheumatoid arthritis, were tested.
3. Some of the ranges of motion are depicted in Figure 2. There was little difference between the normal males and females. Active motion was about 25°. Passive motion was about 30° in the radial direction and more at 36° in the ulnar direction. In the arthritics, the active motion was about half of normal, and the passive motion was strongly biased ulnarward.
4. Some of the values for strength are given in Table 1. The average maximum pinch force which could be applied by males was about 8 kgf, chuck pinch and key pinch where the support was greater giving the higher values. In females, the force was about 6 kgf. The arthritic patients could only exert from 1-2 kgf. Radial and ulnar forces were small compared with those of pinch, and again the arthritics were much weaker than normal, which explains the reduced active radial-ulnar motion. Grip strength was nearly ten times reduced in arthritics. Manipulation times for males, females,

and arthritics were 14.8, 16.8 and 34.4 seconds respectively.

THE FIRST DESIGN OF PROSTHESIS

1. The first prosthesis was called the Vari-Axle. (Ref. 2) (Figure 3) The metacarpal component was made from polyethylene, and had an intramedullary stem, joined to a head portion with a spherical surface. Down the centre of the sphere was a slot to accomodate a metal post projecting from the phalangeal component. This component was made from metal. The two components were linked by a snap-in axle which allowed about 15° of radial and ulnar motion each side at extension, and only a few degrees at 90° of flexion. The load-bearing was between the outside of the sphere and a spherical depression in the phalangeal component.

2. A number of mechanical tests were carried out. (Ref. 2). In a wear test, cycling the motion $\pm$ 22 1/2°, cycling the load up to 13.7 kgf, under Ringer's solution at 40° C, for a million cycles, produced only burnishing of the plastic surface, with no other morphological change. Million cycle tests in cyclic lateral loading at a moment of 12.7 kgf cm, resulted in gradual torsion of the plastic head to nearly 40°: this recovered after the test to leave only 5°-10° of distortion. Pull-out tests on the metal stems cemented into a metallic plate gave forces from 14 to 65 kgf, with a mean of 43 kgf.

3. The Vari-Axle prosthesis was tested clinically in 104 joints, in 31 hands of 28 patients. (Ref. 8) The indications were severe rheumatoid arthritis in 24 hands, the remainder being a variety. Postoperatively the hand was maintained in a compression dressing for 5 days or more. Motion was then started using a dynamic splint for exercise and a resting splint for night-time use.

4. Only patients with a follow up of six months or more were included in the study: two prostheses were removed for infection, and these were not included in the following analysis. That left twenty-four hands in 21 patients, from 6 months to 3 years and a mean time of 15.3 months.

5. The pain relief was good, most patients postoperatively having none or only slight pain. The average active range of motion preoperatively was 33°: this fell to only 22° after the operation, a disappointing result. On the positive side however, while most patients preoperatively had severe or moderate ulnar deviation, postoperatively most had none or moderate deviation. The various types of pinch strength and grip strength were measured using the apparatus described earlier. Pinch strength and the radial and ulnar forces were about 25% of normal and this did not change postoperatively. There was, however, a gain in grip strength to nearly one-third of normal, probably due to the better alignments of the fingers and the more useful functional range of motion.

6. There were four dislocations of the axles in early cases: subsequently the axle design was improved. On radiographic examination, a radioluscent line was noted to occur on one or more components in 18 hands, but there were no clinical manifestations. No fractures of any of the components were evident.

TESTING OF POLYETHYLENE INTRAMEDULLARY STEMS

1. Due to the potential distortions which could occur in polyethylene intramedullary stems, it was considered necessary to construct a machine for rapid and long-term testing. (Ref. 9) A circular stem 5mm in diameter, roughened by machining marks,

was cemented concentrically into an aluminum tube, leaving an annular cement wall 1mm thick. A ball-bearing was placed over the projecting part of the stem and a weight was attached to the bearing. The weight W produced a shearing force W across the plastic stem, as well as a bending moment Wa at the section where the stem entered the cement, 'a' being the distance from the weight to the entry point. The aluminum tube and the plastic stem were rotated at 5 revolutions per second, the weight remaining vertical. Hence, the shear force and the bending moment effectively rotated around the plastic stem. This would simulate the application of forces in a multitude of directions. Failure was arbitrarily chosen as when a point on the projecting plastic stem sagged by a certain distance, at which time the machine was stopped.

2. Table 2 summarises the results. Failure always occurred in the region where the stem entered the cement. There were three phenomena: necking, due to repeated stretching without complete recovery, leading to a reduced area; abrasion, caused by rubbing of the acrylic cement due to micromovements from elastic deformation between the cement and the polyethylene; and cracking, where a fatigue crack developed, sometimes initiated apparently by digging in of the acrylic cement edge into the polyethylene. The bending stresses were clearly more influential than the shear, in causing failure The bending moment at the maximum shear force before failure, 1.13 kgf, was 5.50 kgf cm.

3. Based on these results, it was concluded that if even moderately high forces were applied over the long-term, some failures may occur in polyethylene stems. It was therefore decided that one criterion for the design of a mechanical prosthesis should be to use metallic intramedullary stems.

DESIGN AND EVALUATION OF THE LOAD-STABILISING PROSTHESIS

1. The design of this prosthesis was based on the experience with the Vari-Axle and on further considerations. The prosthesis is shown in Figure 4. The metacarpal and phalangeal components are metal (cast cobalt-chrome alloy), with a plastic insert between. The phalangeal component has a ball on a stem. The stem can accept a shearing force of 22 kgf and a bending moment of 10.8 kgf cm before any bending would occur. Such forces are not expected to occur in the arthritic hand.

2. The plastic insert is based on a cylinder. Across the top of the cylinder, there is a shallow recess in an attempt to provide location for the extensor tendon. It is expected that a cylindrical surface, with the recess, will maintain the extensor tendon at a constant lever arm from the centre of rotation. In contrast, if the metacarpal component were a spherical surface, the tendon could readily align over the side at a reduced lever arm.

3. The intramedullary stems are for cement fixation. To restrain rotation and to provide orientation during insertion there are triangular gussets to be keyed into slots cut into the sides of the prepared bones.

4. The plastic insert is first snapped over the ball of the phalangeal component. The insert is then pressed on to the fork of the metacarpal component, after which the ball cannot escape, because the plastic can no longer expand sideways.

5. An important feature of the prosthesis is that load-bearing occurs between the exterior cylindrical surface of the plastic insert, and the concave cylindrical surface of the phalangeal component.

128

This maximises the surface area. On the large size, the area is 0.74 cm^2, giving a contact stress at maximum pinch force in the male of 86 kgf/cm^2. The stress in a Charnley hip prosthesis at four times body weight is about 72 kgf/cm^2.

6. There is a slight lack of conformity between the cylindrical surfaces, to allow a certain amount of laxity without digging-in of the metal into the plastic. Radial-ulnar linear movement is small. There is about 7 1/2° of radial and ulnar rotation and about 10° of axial rotation built into the prosthesis. When the joint is not loaded, this laxity will allow the finger to have freedom of position and will attenuate any external high forces, which might be applied. As soon as a compressive force is applied however, such as in pinch or grip activities, the cylindrical surfaces align the prosthesis in the flexion-extension plane. This represents stability, and hence the name of the prosthesis.

7. In order to carry out detailed studies of the mechanical behaviour of the Load-Stabilising prosthesis, a machine has been constructed which can simultaneously and independently apply a compressive force, a shear force, and a bending moment to the prosthesis. (Fig. 5) The prosthesis is cemented into metal tubes (or bones) and is rotated at one revolution each two seconds, to cycle the shear force and bending moment. By suitable oriented guides, the bending moment only occurs in the radial-ulnar plane. Obviously the joint cannot accept a moment in the flexion-extension plane, as it would simply collapse.

8. It is of interest to describe the behaviour of the prosthesis under different loading combinations. Assume a compressive load C is first applied. (Fig. 6) The stress distribution across the joint is uniform. Let a moment M, say in the ulnar direction, be slowly applied. The stress on the ulnar side will increase and that on the radial side will decrease. A level of M is reached when tilting just begins to occur about the ulnar corner. The stress at the radial side is zero. It can readily be shown that, assuming a linear elastic system, the moment on the initiation of tilting is given by:

$$M = 1/6 \ a \ C$$

For example, assume that there is a compressive force of 20 kgf acting on a prosthesis which is 1 cm in width, the moment to initiate tilting is 3.3 kgf cm.

9. In fact, the plastic cylindrical surface has been modified slightly to take account of the redistribution of stress due to a moment superimposed on a compressive force. The cylinder has been barrelled, such that the diameter at the extremes is about 1/4mm less than near the centre, and the outer corners have been radiused to prevent distortion.

10. Clinical trials have just begun on this prosthesis at the time of writing (October 1976) and it is expected that reports will be made when sufficient long-term data has been obtained.

REFERENCES

1. DOBYNS, J. H. Total MP joint replacements Surgery of the Upper Extremity in Arthritis. conf. sponsored by American Society for Surgery of the Hand, Hyannis, Mass., Sept. 7-9, 1976.

2. WALKER, P.S. and ERKMAN, M.J. Laboratory evaluation of a metal-plastic type of metacarpophalangeal joint prosthesis. Clinical Orthopaedics, 112, 349, 1975.

3. UNSWORTH A., DOWSON D. and WRIGHT, V. Cracking joints. Ann. rheum. Dis., 30, 348, 1971.

4. ALEKSANDROWICZ R, PAGOWSKI A., and SEYFREID, A. Anatomic-Geometric and kinematic analysis of the MCP joint. Folia Morphol (Warsz), 33, 353, 1974.

5. SWANSON, A.B., MATEV, I.B. and deGROOT, G. The strength of the hand. Inter-Clinic Information Bulletin, 13, 1, 1974.

6. LONG, C., CONRAD, P.W., HALL, E.A., and FURTER, S.L. Intrinsic-Extrinsic muscle control of the hand in power grip and precision handling. J Bone and Joint Surg., 52A, 853, 1970.

7. DICKSON, R.A., and NICOLLE, F. V. The assessment of hand function, The Hand, 8, 110, 1976.

8. MONEIM, M.S., and STRAUB, L.S., JR. Clinical evaluation of a cemented prosthesis in the MCP joint. Private communication of prepared paper, Hospital for Special Surgery.

9. DIAMOND, R, WALKER, P.S., and NOVICK, G. Plastic intramedullary stems for prosthetic components, Proc. 23rd Annual Orthopaedic Research Society, Las Vegas, Feb. 1-3, 1976

	MALE	FEMALE	ARTHRITIC FEMALE
Pulp pinch, index	7.5	5.7	1.3
Pulp pinch, long	6.6	5.0	1.1
Lateral pinch, index	8.2	5.7	1.2
Chuck pinch	8.7	6.7	1.4
Key pinch	9.2	7.4	2.0
Radial force, index	1.78	1.06	0.18
Ulnar force, index	1.49	0.81	0.24
Grip strength	15.6	8.1	0.9

Table 1
Average maximum strength values (kilograms force)

SHEAR FORCE (kgf)	BENDING STRESS (kgf/cm^2)	MILLIONS OF CYCLES TO NO FAILURE OR TO FAILURE (F)
0.45	86	4.5,4.4,4.6,4.4,4.4,4.4,7.5,7.5
0.68	134	5.7,5.7,6.4,5.7,5.7
0.91	179	5.4,4.6,5.0,4.0,4.8,2.5,4.2,2.5
1.13	224	5.0,5.1,5.0,5.0,2.2,2.5,2.5,F
1.36	269	4.6,4.8,3.5,4.0,F,F,F,F
1.59	314	5.4,4.2,F,F,F
1.81	358	1.3,F,F,F,F

Table 2
The results of long-term rotating shear and
bending tests on cemented polyethylene stems.

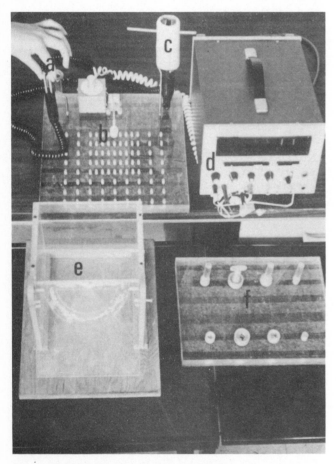

Fig. 1: The apparatus for evaluating the hand.
a pinch forces b radial and ulnar forces c grip forces
d digit strain recorder e radial and ulnar movement at
different flexion angles f manipulative ability

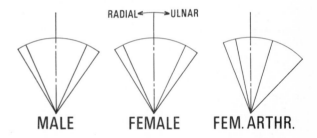

Fig. 2: Ranges of ulnar and radial motion (drawn to scale) for
the index finger at 0° flexion

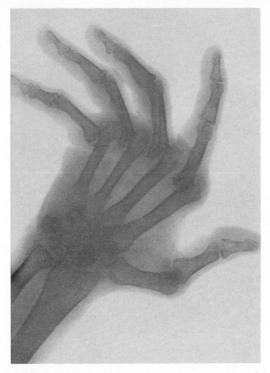
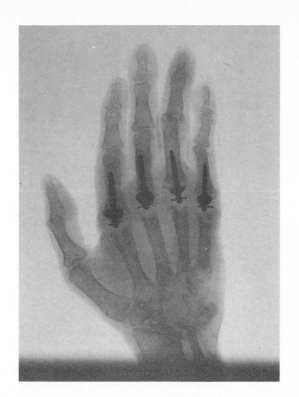

Fig. 3: Radiographs of a typical case in which the Vari-Axle prosthesis was clinically evaluated

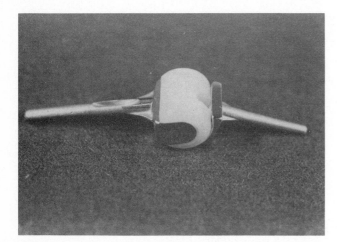
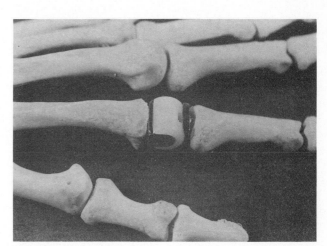

Fig. 4: The load-stabilizing MCP prosthesis

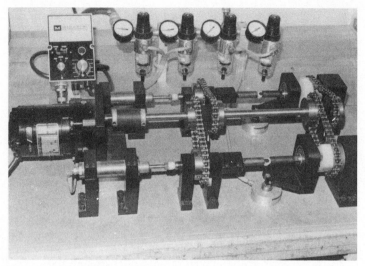

Fig. 5 Two-channel finger prosthesis test machine. A compressive force, shear force, and a radial-moment can be applied independently

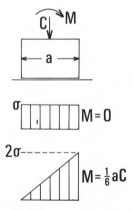

Fig. 6: The stress distribution on the cylindrical bearing surface when a compressive force C is applied (top) and when a radial or ulnar moment M=1/6 a C is superimposed to just initiate tilting

MODIFIED DESIGN OF ENCAPSULATED METACARPO-PHALANGEAL JOINT PROSTHESIS FOR THE RHEUMATOID HAND

F. NICOLLE, MChir, FRCS,
Royal Postgraduate Medical School, Ducane Road, Hammersmith, London

Introduction:

We have now reached a stage where time and experience has allowed hand surgeons to judge for themselves the true merit of current designs of finger joint prostheses. We are all familiar with the shortcomings of the prosthetic materials available. No plastic is indestructable; silicone rubber fractures more readily after implantation than under simulated bench testing. Polypropylene is more durable, but as an integral hinge, it is insufficiently strong to withstand more vigorous manual movement, which creates excessive compression and tortional stress. The purpose of today's presentation is to demonstrate our current design of a modified finger joint, and the results obtained since its introduction into clinical use in October 1974.

The original design of an encapsulated polypropylene hinge joint has been employed since the beginning of 1970, and a recent study (Griffiths and Nicolle 1975) published in 1975, showed the results obtained after an average follow-up period of twenty months. These results showed the following complications in a total of 112 joints replaced (Table 1). In our experience, we have also had a few cases of hinge fracture, but this did not occur in the cases studied.

The prosthesis was well tolerated with a very low incidence of infection or foreign body reaction, but the incidence of capsular fracture was felt to be unacceptably high, although this most often had no adverse effect on finger joint function. These results, and the experience of other surgeons with different prostheses, have prompted us to try to evolve an improved design

The incidence of capsular fracture is closely similar to that of silicone prostheses and emphasises the limited durability of this material, if subjected to repeated compression and flexion. In our design, the capsule provides both a desirable soft cushion between the tendons and the hinge, as well as sealing off dead space and preventing fibrous tissue ingrowth during wound healing.

The original polypropylene hinge has been replaced by a much stronger partially constrained cylindrical bearing of clinical grade stainless steel, fitting into a socket of polypropylene. This hinge permits an unlimited range of flexion and extension, but beyond 180 degrees extension, the bearing begins to dislocate, although it remains stable for a further 35 degrees.

Similarly, when flexed to less than 90 degrees it dislocates, but remains stable for a further 20 degrees. The clyindrical bearing has ends which are slightly bevelled into a convex form, which allows a passive range of sideways mobility of 15 degrees on either side of a straight line. The hinge mechanism shows acceptable tolerance to wear under laboratory conditions, and provides a much stronger and yet semi-constrained design compared with an integral hinge of silicone or polypropylene. A hinge measurement which provides a stable fulcrum for flexion movement is likely also to contribute to a stronger pinch force in the post-operative result.

The intramedullary stems were redesigned with four flanges in order to resist rotation in the bone, and thus to improve finger stability.

The prostheses are made in six different sizes, and furthermore, the proximal and distal ends of the four small sizes can be interchanged, if circumstances require this, in order to gain a more accurate fit in the intramedullary canals.

After reaming out the bone ends, a set of colour coded Sizers are used to determine the appropriate size of joint prosthesis. The prostheses are pre-sterilized in packets ready for immediate use.

Clinical Results:

Since October 1974, 82 of these new design of prostheses have been used in 20 patients (Table 2). The clinical results have been generally better than with the previous prostheses. The incidence of complications (Table 3) showed a striking improvement in the durability of the prostheses, but a slight increase in the rate of infection. This latter feature may well reflect an undue relaxing of our standards of technique, and the fact that the operative procedure, which is an exacting one, is now being done by surgeons of less experience in our surgical unit.

All cases were included in an ongoing study to assess levels of pre and post-operative deformity, flexion force, grip strength and the range of movement. Unfortunately, not all cases could be included in the final analysis, since a number have returned overseas, or been lost in follow-up. However, 53 joint replacements were available for this current assessment. The results given today require longer follow-up and additional numbers, before they can be regarded as significant statistically, but I do not feel that this precludes the value of a preliminary report at this time.

Subjective assessment showed a generally very high level of patient satisfaction, but our main concern was to determine the long term benefit, if any, in terms of increased flexion force at the digital level, and the incidence, if any, of recurrent deformity, particularly ulnar drift at the meta-carpo-phalangeal joints.

These results are summarised in the following two tables, and again, it is stressed that on a strict statistical level, these are not yet significant.

Table 4 shows flexion force in the digits (Dixon and Nicolle 1972) where the metacarpo-phalangeal joints have been replaced in 53 digits. There are fewer cases available for long term follow-up, and a further assessment in a year's time will be a valuable contribution. It does, however, appear from comparison of the twelve month and twenty-four month periods of follow-up, that the degree of improvement is well maintained. It would be informative to know which of these cases had experienced an exacerbation of their arthritis during the period of follow-up, as this undoubtedly would contribute to deterioration, which might otherwise be blamed on the operative procedure.

Table 5 shows the degree of ulnar drift (Irregbulam and Nicolle 1974) measured pre-operatively and during the two-year period of follow-up. It is plotted as the average change in ulnar drift of all the joints available at each period of assessment. It can be clearly seen that ulnar drift was not only improved by surgery, but appears to decrease further with progressive rehabilitation of the hand post-operatively. The latter is most probably related to improved muscle power and balance, and emphasises the importance of supervised exercises and dynamic splinting during the post-operative period.

However, from twelve months onwards, we see progressive drift, for which the reason is not yet clear. Again, we need to know more of the medical condition of the patient, and whether exacerbation or general deteriotation is the underlying cause of this change. Our clinical impression is that this ulnar deviation of up to an average of 18 degrees does not adversely affect hand function.

Conclusion:

Trick movements and ingenuity enable patients with gross hand deformity to function surprisingly well, and therefore, standardised methods of assessment tend to be rather artificial. The evolution of improved finger joint prostheses comes through a combination of long-term clinical observation and objective assessment. Likewise, the assessment of this new design requires to be measured in the long term, and today's data must serve as an interim report. We can, however, see evidence of improved durability of the prostheses, as well as indications of a more sustained improvement in hand function.

REFERENCES

1. Griffiths R.W. and Nicolle F.V. (1975): "Three years experience of metacarpo-phalangeal joint replacement in the rheumatoid hand". The Hand, 7, 275 - 283.

2. Dixon R.A. and Nicolle F.V. (1972): "The assessment of hand function Part 1". The Hand, 4, 207 - 214.

3. Irregbulam L.M., Nicolle F.V., and Calnan J.C. (1974): "Measurement of digital deviation. A simple device". The Hand, 6, 166 - 171.

Total	112
Capsular fracture	31
Shaft fracture	5
Hinge fracture	0
Hinge dislocation	6
Early infection	1
Late infection	1

Table 1
Complications — original joint prosthesis

Average follow-up	12 months
Prostheses inserted	82
Prostheses available for follow-up	53
Sex Female 18 Male	2
Average age	56
Sero positive	16
Mean duration of disease	17 years

Table 2
M.C.P. joint replacement

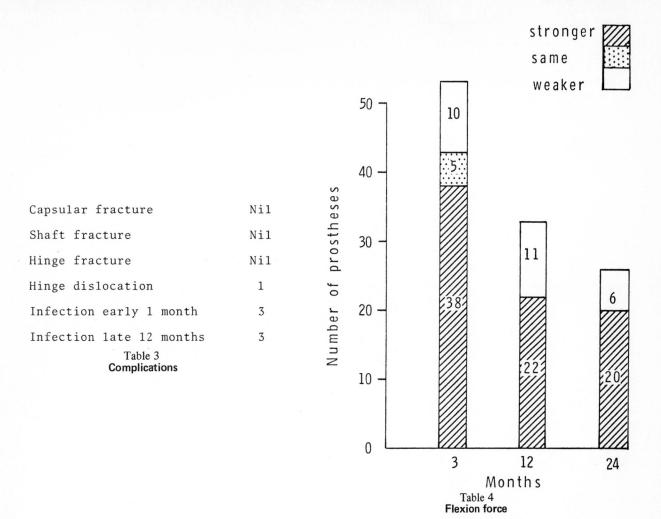

Capsular fracture	Nil
Shaft fracture	Nil
Hinge fracture	Nil
Hinge dislocation	1
Infection early 1 month	3
Infection late 12 months	3

Table 3
Complications

Table 4
Flexion force

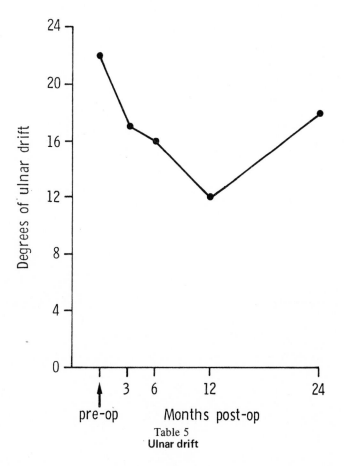

Table 5
Ulnar drift